SO, YOU WANT TO BE A DOCTOR, EH?

So, You Want to be a Doctor, Eh?

A Guidebook to Canadian Medical School

Dr. Anne Berndl, M.D.

**Part of the Writing on Stone
Canadian Career Series**

Writing on Stone Press
PO Box 259, Raymond, AB T0K 2S0
(403) 752-4800
www.writingonstone.ca

Published by:
Writing on Stone Press Inc.
P.O. Box 259
Raymond, Alberta, Canada T0K 2S0
(403) 752-4800
Fax: (403) 752-4815
Email: info@writingonstone.ca
Web: http://www.writingonstone.ca

**LIBRARY AND ARCHIVES CANADA
CATALOGUING IN PUBLICATION**

Berndl, Anne, 1980-
So, You Want to be a Doctor, Eh? : A Guidebook to Canadian
Medical School / Anne Berndl.

(Writing on Stone Canadian Career Series)
ISBN 978-0-9781309-0-9

1. Physicians--Vocational guidance--Canada. 2. Medical
education--Canada. 3. Medical colleges--Canada. I. Title.
II. Series.

R749.A6B473 2007   610.71'171   C2007-905195-2

To my family, who told me to reach for the stars,
and to Murray, who makes it all possible.

CONTENTS

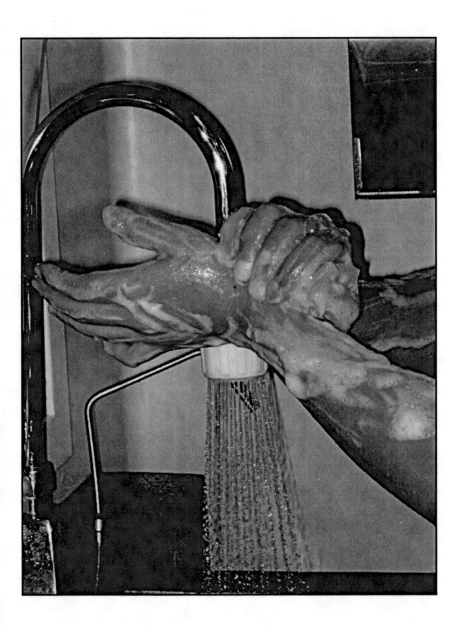

FOREWORD:

YOU may wonder if you need a book about obtaining a medical education. I assure you that you do, and that this is the one, particularly if you are considering practicing medicine in Canada. This book is uniquely Canadian, offering a comprehensive guide to navigating the process of becoming a physician in Canada today. In a country where there are far fewer training positions than applicants, this book provides useful statistics, application tips, and wonderful narratives from individuals involved in every step of the medical training journey.

Whether medicine has been a lifelong dream, or like me, another component of an established career path, this book will help you to consider the personal, intellectual, physical, and financial challenges along the very long road of medical training. As you read this book, you will be encouraged to make thoughtful decisions based on self-awareness and careful reflections on the many exciting career opportunities that exist in the medical field.

I have counselled hundreds of post-secondary students with personal, career, and academic struggles prior to studying medicine, and I believe that the best career decisions are made when you know yourself, know your options, and make informed decisions that are your own. The practise of medicine is stimulating and filled with opportunities to help and heal people that will bring you feelings of incredible joy and satisfaction; however, medical training is rigorous and perpetually challenging, and at times, amazingly difficult. As such, it is crucial to make sure that a career in medicine is for you.

Reading this book is a great start to making an informed decision about a medical career. Becoming acquainted with career planning resources at your school is another way to gather useful information. Many colleges and universities offer career counselling and career planning workshops, which can help to determine if medicine will suit you. Information is the key to successful career planning, so consider conducting informational interviews with medical students, residents, and practising physicians to find out what they consider to be the realities– the best *and* worst aspects– of their careers.

No matter where you are in the process of considering or obtaining a medical education, this book can help you face the challenges at each stage of the process. A career in medicine affords extraordinary possibilities to those who choose it, but it is a long, tough journey– so consider it carefully, and ultimately decide to do what is most inspiring and meaningful to you.

Dr. Sherry James, M.D., M.Ed., BA.
Psychiatry Resident, Dalhousie University

PART I:
INTRODUCTION
TO MEDICINE

CHAPTER 1: ABOUT THIS BOOK

Why I Wrote This Book

THE road to becoming a doctor is long. Even the shortest path requires eight additional years of education beyond high school. The majority of doctors are educated between ten and fifteen years beyond their high school education before they can practice medicine independently. The initial step of getting into medical school requires jumping through a number of prescribed hoops, while at the same time maintaining your individuality.

When I started to consider medicine as a career, I had no real references to guide me. There were many books targeted towards American "premeds," but resources that would help organize my application to Canadian schools were not available, and so I had to discover and research each step of the road myself. The year I applied to medical school I was also writing a 4th year thesis and getting married. It would have decreased my stress levels significantly if there had been a guide available that would have walked me through the process, given me advice, and offered me insight into the process of becoming a physician. I later decided to create a webpage (http://www.drstarter.ca) to fulfill this need, and it has since evolved into this book.

The information I'm sharing with you is from my personal experiences and the experiences of other medical students and residents who have where you are now. If there is a theme in this book, it's to maintain a sense of self and persevere. Good luck to you - this is a road worth traveling, O future physician!

What Qualifies Me to Write This Book?

Like you, I'm a real person who had a real dream. I did not come from a family of well-established physicians who could help me along the way, so I did a lot of reading and researching on my own to find out about the process of applying to medical school. I didn't make this choice lightly—prior to applying I spent a lot of time ensuring this was what I wanted to do. I probably went a little overboard, but I felt that I needed to know what I was getting into. Since I started my residency, I have often been asked what it's like to be a doctor, what medical school was like, and how others should go about pursuing the same career path.

I've been there. I've suffered through organic chemistry and the MCAT. I searched for and was able to find volunteer activities that challenged and inspired me. I spent hours editing, reading, and perfecting my applications, and I want to share these experiences with you. The journey is long but the reward is sweet. I'll never forget the first time I really connected with a patient, delivered my first baby, or was handed the knife to open a belly for the first time.

Many of my colleagues, medical students, and residents have also contributed their insight to this book. There's definitely no single path to becoming a doctor, and I hope the variety of opinions and experiences will help you to find your own way. I sincerely hope this book helps you to organize yourself throughout the application process and the medical school and residency experiences. I hope to give you optimism with a dose of reality. Good luck to you!

Thanks to Those Who Contributed

I'd like to thank the following people who gave their thoughtful insight and time, allowed me to interview them for this book, and provided samples of their applications:

Dr. Sandra de Montbrun;
Dr. Rickesh Sood;
Dr. Jennifer Graham;
Dr. Christopher McCrossin;
Dr. Midori Yamamoto;

Dr. Allison Ball;

Dr. Alon Altman;

The Soon To-Be Dr. Alia Mukhiah;

and

Dr. Sherry James, who kindly used her expertise as a previous career counsellor to write the foreword to this book.

The Ultimate Canadian Medical School Resource Guide: What Sets This Book Apart?

Currently, if you're a Canadian interested in getting into medical school, the information at your disposal is directed towards American students. These books may provide a general idea about what getting into medical school requires, but they are also packed full of information that does not apply to you as a prospective Canadian student. Canada does not have any explicitly "premed" undergraduate programs, and there are no undergraduate premed advisors to write letters of recommendation for you. No programs exist that give conditional offers out of high school outside of Quebec. There are more applicants per available medical school seat in Canada. For these reasons, getting into medical school in Canada is more difficult than it is in the United States. The back-up plans available to Canadians are also different, as doing medical school in a foreign country carries many greater challenges for a Canadian than for an American, and Canada does not have positions such as a "doctor's assistant" as a realistic alternative career.

There have been other books published about Canadian medical schools, but they tend to focus on statistics and minimum GPAs - information that can be useful but limited. This book is comprehensive and goes beyond the information you'll find on every medical schools' home page. My aim is to provide a clear outline of the challenges you'll face as you prepare for, apply to, and succeed in medical school. This book will not only show you how to get where you're going, but will show you what you're getting yourself into. It's all here: considering medicine as a career, how to spend your time preparing yourself for medicine, getting through the MCAT and the interviews, and preparing back-up plans. Information about the medical school experience and life as a resident has also been included. I hope these sections give you a glimpse of the medical world you are hoping to become part of, so that you can better prepare yourself for this endeavour. I have compiled current statistics and admission information on all English-speaking medical schools in Canada, so you will know what you need to do to be considered a competitive applicant. I've also spent countless hours interviewing my colleagues to give you a better sense of what this career choice entails. Becoming a doctor takes time and perseverance, and I hope my colleagues' contributions will help give those of you who may be ready to give up a little hope, and help those who may be considering a career in medicine for the wrong reasons reach this same conclusion. This book's thorough exploration of becoming a doctor in Canada is what sets it apart in its field.

CHAPTER 2: INTRODUCTION TO THE JOURNEY

The Road to Becoming a Physician, a Brief Outline

"The life so short, the craft so long to learn."
—*Hippocrates*

MOST physicians are well-rounded people who also excel in academics. They tend to have significant experiences in the arts, athletics, leadership, travel, and volunteer work, as well as maintaining good grades. The thing that sets physicians apart from other science-based careers is the intensive level of interpersonal skills that are required on a daily basis.

The time-line:

High School: 4 years
  Goals:
  ✓ Get good grades
  ✓ Take Grade 12 Biology, Physics, Chemistry, Calculus, and English. These are prerequisites for the university courses you'll later take in order to be eligible for medical school. Make sure you also take courses that interest you such as drama, history, or music.
  ✓ Participate in extracurricular activities and branch out to develop your skills to become a well-rounded person. Enjoy sports, artistic endeavours, volunteer work,

leadership roles, and seek out unique educational opportunities. Participate in the community.

University: 3-4 years
Goals:
- ✓ Maintain your high grades
- ✓ Write the MCAT
- ✓ Continue to participate in activities you started in high school, while taking on additional responsibility
- ✓ Apply to medical school

Medical School: 3-4 years
Goals:
- ✓ Pre-clerkship
- ✓ Clerkship
- ✓ Continue some extracurricular activities
- ✓ Choose a specialty
- ✓ Apply for residency
- ✓ Write the Medical Council of Canada Qualifying Examination (MCCQE) Part I
- ✓ Graduate with an M.D.
- ✓ Congratulations! You're now a Doctor!
- ✓ Over 97% of students who start medical school finish medical school.
  (http://umanitoba.ca/faculties/medicine/admissions/info.html)

Residency: 2-6 years
Goals:
- ✓ Survive PGY1 (Post Graduate Year One, the internship year)
- ✓ Write the MCCQE part II
- ✓ Increase your level of knowledge and independence with each passing year
- ✓ Write the licensing exam for your area of specialty
- ✓ Start work in your area of specialty
- ✓ Or, apply for fellowships

Fellowship or Extra Training: 3 months-3 years
Goals:
- ✓ Write your fellowship exams
- ✓ Begin looking for work in your sub-specialized field

If you start thinking about medicine at the beginning of high school, and if you take the shortest route possible, the minimum amount of time between grade 9 and becoming an independent family physician is twelve years. Many people either do not apply after their undergraduate degree or are not accepted after their undergraduate degree. These people are still eligible to apply while working or taking additional schooling, as long as the minimum three to four years of undergraduate education has been completed.

What Do Doctors Do?

There are many opportunities available to doctors. In general, doctors prevent, discuss, diagnose, and treat disease— both medically and surgically. They also educate in the area of health, conduct medical science research, teach other doctors and students, communicate honestly about complex and emotional topics with patients and families, advocate on behalf of their patients, and provide emotional support and information to people who are ill. Doctors monitor and support the biological, psychological, and social health of their patients, and often manage teams of healthcare providers.

Doctors work in hospitals, clinics, and sometimes in people's homes. Physicians have the opportunity to meet unique groups of people: they can volunteer at rural clinics oversees or local clinics for the homeless, they can teach in a university, or they can travel abroad to participate in international conferences.

Physicians work long and unorthodox hours. When a resident says they have a teaching session at six o'clock, it could just as easily be at six at night at six in the morning. Doctors often come in on weekends to round on patients in the hospital, and carry a pager with them so they can be contacted. It's not uncommon to work ten- to twelve-hour days without an opportunity to sit down and eat. The average physician works fifty hours per week, excluding time spent on call.[1]

---

[1] *National Physician Survey* [http://www.cfpc.ca/nps/English/home.asp]. College of Family Physicians of Canada, Canadian Medical Association,

Most physicians are on call in some form, be it in-house, where they must stay overnight at the hospital, or home where they may be called back to see a patient at any time. When doctors are on call, it is likely they have worked the day before, often resulting in staying awake for twenty-four to thirty-six hours in a row. Medical students and residents are generally on call one day of every four, whereas actual staff are on call much less often, or at least do more on-call work from home instead of in-house.

There are mundane parts to a physician's day. There are forms to fill, charts to dictate, phone calls to answer, blood work to go through and sign. As a medical student and resident, especially in the earlier years, you'll find yourself doing a lot of form-filling and discharge summaries. This type of work is generally called "scut"—it has to be done and no one likes it.

Doctors are often quite involved in their communities. Many doctors volunteer their time to both medical and non-medical causes. They can speak with authority about issues that affect people's health, such as pesticide use and wearing bicycle helmets. They can also become involved on a political level to make changes.

Doctors are doctors both inside and outside the hospital. Since becoming a doctor, I've treated a broken finger in Costa Rica, a broken arm on a ski hill, an allergic reaction on an airplane, and have done CPR on the side of the road after a car had a head-on collision with a moose. Your skills will be portable, universal, and needed.

As a physician, you will be present at defining moments in people's lives. You'll witness births and deaths—often participating intimately in the event. You'll see people at their strongest and weakest moments, which are amazingly, often the same. You'll be confronted with intense emotions; there will be days where you will feel like a healer and days where you will feel you can do nothing and are helpless. You'll be asked daily to make hard decisions, to explain complex matters, and to respect choices that may differ from your own. You'll feel like there's not enough time to do everything that's asked of you, but at the same time, you'll be discouraged from hurrying. You'll have patients who are mean, kind, self-righteous,

Royal College of Physicians and Surgeons of Canada; 2004. Accessed 2007 July. Available from: www.nationalphysiciansurvey.ca.

giving, afraid, complacent, strong, wonderful, and inspiring. It will be your daily challenge to achieve trust, get to the heart of the matter, and provide care accordingly.

CanMed Guidelines

These are the guidelines by which physicians are judged. They must be competent in all areas presented in order to successfully complete residency. This list will give you an idea of the skills required of a physician, along with several examples of each.

Medical Expert
- ✓ Knowing the potential side effects of a medication
- ✓ Knowing how to diagnose strep throat
- ✓ Being able to palpate the liver
- ✓ Performing an appendectomy

Communicator
- ✓ Sensing that someone is uncomfortable with a treatment plan and finding out why
- ✓ Listening patiently to an ill person and empathising with their fears
- ✓ Explaining a complex medical concept to someone clearly enough for them to make an informed decision
- ✓ Providing information to a team of health professionals so they can collaborate or continue care

Collaborator
- ✓ Working with a team. Recognising distinct expert roles and respecting these roles
- ✓ Asking for help from appropriate people when needed

Manager
- ✓ Being a team leader
- ✓ Being aware of available resources and using them effectively
- ✓ Using time effectively

Health Advocate
- ✓ Standing up for something in which you believe

✓ Finding a cause and working on its behalf
✓ Trying to change a wrong you've observed
✓ Being aware of the multifactorial issues that contribute to health
✓ Understanding and advocating prevention

Scholar

✓ Participating in research
✓ Expressing a desire to go deeper into a topic
✓ Taking an interest in the learning opportunities available to you
✓ Teaching others

Professional

✓ Being accountable for your actions
✓ Trying to right your wrongs
✓ Being honest, compassionate, respectful of privacy, and owning up to your responsibilities

Residency Positions Available in Canada 2006

The following are residency positions that may be available after completing medical school. This list is not an extensive list of the types of doctors in Canada—merely a list of residency positions that are available immediately following medical school. In addition to the following list of residency programs, there are further periods of training that some doctors complete, known as a fellowship, which allows them to sub-specialize in a particular field. For example, a vascular surgeon would complete the general surgery residency, and then continue with a fellowship in vascular surgery. Cardiologists would start in internal medicine and then apply for a cardiology fellowship. Neonatologists would begin in a paediatric residency and then fellowship in neonatology.

Anatomical Pathology: Examining specimens and diagnosing illnesses based on tissue and cell samples, conducting autopsies.

Anaesthesia: Caring for patients whether they are unconscious or awake during surgery, helping patients manage pain, intubating patients, and putting in lines.

Cardiac Surgery: Operating on the heart, replacing valves, bypassing clogged arteries.

Community medicine: Looking at the health of a community as a whole, preventative care.

Dermatology: Treating conditions of the skin, rashes, cancers, moles.

Diagnostic Radiology: Interpreting X-rays, ultrasounds, MRIs, CT scans. Interventional Radiologists perform micro-procedures under the guidance of imaging.

Emergency medicine: Treating patients who present to the emergency department, the initial contact person for patients with any problem that causes them to go to the hospital.

Family medicine: Caring for patients and their families on a long-term basis. Developing a relationship with patients and providing primary care for them during their lifespan.

General pathology: Examining specimens and diagnosing illnesses based on tissue and cell samples.

General Surgery: Performing surgery on organs of the abdomen such as bowel surgery, appendectomies, hernia repairs, pancreatic and gall bladder surgeries. They also remove masses from soft tissues in the body.

Haematological Pathology: Examining and making diagnoses based on blood and marrow samples, overseeing blood transfusions and acting as a consultant to determine which tests are best used to diagnose an illness.

Internal medicine: treating patients with diseases of the organs such as heart attacks, lung cancer, liver disease, diabetes and kidney problems. They can be treated either with medication or invasive procedures. Subspecialties include (but are not limited to) cardiology, endocrinology, gerontology, nephrology, and rheumatology.

Laboratory Medicine: A discipline that often encompasses anatomical pathology, general pathology, and medical microbiology.

Medical Genetics: Counseling patients with genetic-based diseases such as cancers, metabolic diseases, and birth defects.

Medical Microbiology: Using lab skills to investigate and treat infections. Controlling outbreaks and being consulted on complex cases of infection.

Neurology: Diagnosing and treating diseases of the nervous system such as stroke, Alzheimer's, and Multiple Sclerosis.

Paediatric Neurology: Diagnosing and treating diseases of the nervous system in children such as epilepsy and cerebral palsy.

Neurosurgery: Operating on the brain and nervous system and treating cases such as head trauma, cancers of the nervous system, and spinal injuries.

Nuclear Medicine: Using dynamic imaging to diagnose clinical problems, this physiologic imaging can be applied to almost every branch of medicine.

Obstetrics and Gynaecology: Medical and surgical treatment of diseases of the female reproductive tract and bladder as well as caring for women during pregnancy.

Occupational Medicine: Treating and preventing work-related disorders such as limb injuries and asthma. Research into workplace health and advocating for safer work areas.

Ophthalmology: Medical and surgical treatment of diseases of the eye.

Orthopaedic Surgery: Performing surgery on bones such as knees, shoulders and spines.

Otolaryngology: Surgical treatment of ears, noses, and throats.

Paediatrics: Diagnosing and treating illness in children.

Physical Therapy and Rehabilitation: Using physiotherapy to treat musculoskeletal and neurological disease to help patients achieve their highest potential of rehabilitation.

Plastic Surgery: Surgically treating burns and other damage to hands and faces, including reconstructive surgery.

Psychiatry: Diagnosing and treating mental illnesses such as depression, schizophrenia, bipolar disorder, and anxiety.

Radiation Oncology: Overseeing the use of radiation as a treatment for cancer.

Urology: Surgically treating diseases of the kidney, uriters, prostate, and bladder.

Who Becomes an M.D. in Canada?

Medical students come from a variety of backgrounds and experiences. Medical students are teachers, lawyers, and computer engineers. The majority of them have completed a four-year science degree, but there are also those from midwifery, music, and math backgrounds. About half of them decided they wanted to be doctors before or during high school.[2] Among medical students, there are a variety of past experiences, talents and abilities, and different languages spoken. If you're eavesdropping on a group of medical students discussing their lives prior to entering the field of medicine, you are likely to overhear a conversation about previously managing a bar, skating professionally, traveling to Haiti or being pregnant with a second child.

The average newly-admitted medical student is twenty-four years old, but students as old as forty-three have received admission.[3] Most

---

[2] *National Physician Survey* [http://www.cfpc.ca/nps/English/home.asp]. College of Family Physicians of Canada, Canadian Medical Association, Royal College of Physicians and Surgeons of Canada; 2004. Accessed 2007 July. Medical Student Questionnaire. Available from: www.nationalphysiciansurvey.ca.
[3] *National Physician Survey* [http://www.cfpc.ca/nps/English/home.asp]. College of Family Physicians of Canada, Canadian Medical Association,

medical students have a four-year degree, but some have completed only three years, and still others have PhDs or have spent time working at another job.

Doctors tend to run in families - 15.6% of medical students have a physician parent, (*A. Dahalla et al, CMAJ 2002; 166(8) 1029-35)* and 54% of medical students grew up in an urban setting. According to the 2004 National Physician Survey, 68% of medical school students have at least a bachelor's degree, 10% have a master's degree, 3% have earned a doctorate, and 27% of students in medical school have completed CEGEP.[4] Many applicants have completed four years of post-secondary schooling, but this can range from a single year (if attended CEGEP) to over ten years.

People who are accepted into medical school have A's in the majority of their university courses, and get 10's on average in each of the sections of the MCAT. Medical students have demonstrated that they are skilled socially, academically, and emotionally. They tend to enjoy taking on leadership roles, are comfortable being responsible for the decisions they make, and are extremely self-motivated.

Doc Talk

I think that becoming a doctor has always been at the back of my mind. It wasn't so much the science, but it was seeing the anatomy and looking at the organs from the inside that really intrigued me. I remember being in Jr. high school and there was a "don't smoke" program, and someone brought in a human lung. And I was so delighted by it. I remember one of my friends saying, "Midori, you should be a doctor!"

—*Midori Yamamoto, 4th year medical student*

Royal College of Physicians and Surgeons of Canada; 2004. Accessed 2007 July. Medical Student Questionnaire. Available from: www.nationalphysiciansurvey.ca
[4] When totalled, the actual percentages exceed 100% due to those students who carry multiple degrees

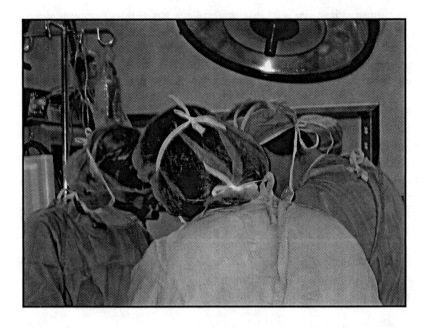

I started out thinking that I was going to ride horses for a living. I rode horses every day after school throughout high school, and most of university. I took a year off after 2nd year and went to Switzerland to ride, went back to school for a year, and then went to Florida for a year to ride. It was while I was in Florida that I was watching a commercial for Doctors Without Borders and I was really intrigued by it. I thought about it more and more as the year went on, and I saw myself doing emergency and international health.

–Christopher McCrossin, 4th year medical student

I decided to be a doctor while I was in high school. I always liked sciences and felt I could apply it best in medicine. I probably knew around grade eleven or twelve. After I decided that I geared everything towards applying to medicine. I didn't have any family members who were in medicine, so I don't really know where the idea came from. I always liked watching The Learning Channel and The Operation - I watched it all the time and loved it. I always loved dissecting.

–Dr. Sandra de Montbrun, 3rd year general surgery resident

I decided to go into medicine later than most. I was already working and I had an arts degree. I was thinking maybe I would go into

constitutional law. I was in teachers' college for a short period of
time, then I did international development for three years.
I worked in public health, which is where I became interested in
medicine. People would come to me with symptoms, and I couldn't
help them. I started thinking it would be nice to have a specific skill
set.

There was a doctor from Winnipeg who was in Laos when I was
there, and one day over dinner she asked, "So, what next?" I was
thinking of traveling to India, and she said, "Well, why not
medicine?" I laughed and said, "Well, I'd never get in!"
Before that, it never really hit me that I wanted to get in but didn't
think I could. But I decided that if I wanted to do it, I really should
try to do it.

—Jennifer Graham, 1ˢᵗ year paediatrics resident

CHAPTER 3: ARE YOU RIGHT FOR MEDICINE AND IS MEDICINE RIGHT FOR YOU?

Pros and Cons of Medicine

Pros:

- ✓ Meet new people everyday
- ✓ Challenging
- ✓ Will always be a need for doctors
- ✓ There's an area of specialty to suit almost every type of personality
- ✓ The opportunity is often available to solve problems
- ✓ You'll save lives and make a true difference in the quality of the lives of others
- ✓ Adrenaline
- ✓ Sense of purpose
- ✓ Amazing human stories
- ✓ Fractal experience of life; from cells, to individuals, to communities
- ✓ Opportunities for travel
- ✓ Opportunities for research
- ✓ Ability to teach and pass on your knowledge to patients, medical students, and younger trainees
- ✓ Feel needed
- ✓ Utilize technical skills
- ✓ Expand on yourself socially, intellectually, emotionally, and technically
- ✓ Powerful, raw human interactions

- ✓ Use new technologies
- ✓ Constantly expanding your view of the world
- ✓ Sense of accomplishment
- ✓ Respected opinion
- ✓ The ability to act in an emergency
- ✓ Sharing with people in times of pain and healing

Cons:

- ✓ Training is long, hard, and exhausting
- ✓ Likely go into substantial debt that will take years to pay
- ✓ Much more paper work than you would expect
- ✓ Family and friends can easily be neglected or delayed if extra effort is not made
- ✓ You will at some point make a mistake that prevents you from sleeping
- ✓ Litigious culture - you'll be sued sometime during your career while trying to help someone
- ✓ Money is not as good as you might think, considering the number of hours worked
- ✓ Frustration at not being able to help some people
- ✓ Someone always needs to be available to patients; patients get sick on big holidays or during important celebrations and this type of work cannot always be put off until tomorrow.
- ✓ Daily risk of violent patients, exposure to infectious agents and body fluids, fear of bringing infection home to your family
- ✓ Working in a medical system can sometimes prevent you from providing the care you'd like to for your patients; proper care and staff may not always be available to you
- ✓ Very high expectations of you both in and out of the medical environment (you'll be judged on how you hold your utensils while eating dinner)
- ✓ High levels of divorce, depression, suicide, drug abuse, and addiction
- ✓ Emotionally very stressful; you'll be exposed to death, pain, and suffering

Doc Talk

The reality is that you're not able to spend as much time with your patients as you'd like. You hear about it all the time, but actually experiencing it, and feeling that frustration...I wish that everyone applying to medicine could feel that before applying and committing themselves. It's funny that people who are applying to medicine are applying because of what they think medicine is, but this is not necessarily based on experience. They may be applying to an idealized idea of medicine, but it's hard to know what it's like until you're actually there.

—Midori Yamamoto, 4th year medical student

Reasons to Become a Doctor, Reasons Not to Become a Doctor

Everyone has different reasons for becoming a doctor, and those reasons are frequently hard to articulate. It often comes down to a sense of purpose or vocation. This is, of course, not an extensive list.

Reasons to Become a Doctor:

✓ Intellectual challenge
✓ Social/emotional challenge
✓ Wanting to make an impact on people's lives
✓ Enjoy challenging leadership positions
✓ Feeling of fulfilling a vocation
✓ Personal contact with individuals
✓ Variety of human interactions
✓ Life-long learning opportunities
✓ Enjoyment of scientific discovery
✓ Enjoy being in charge or managing

Doc Talk

No matter how overwhelmed you might feel with various problems that need to be solved in the world, in medicine you can work with one person at a time, so even making a difference to one person is something that I feel is very valuable.

–Midori Yamamoto, 4th year medical student

Just as there are many good reasons to pursue medicine, there are also many bad ones. Being a doctor is an amazing job, but it requires great personal sacrifice. It requires endurance and carries with it many responsibilities. If any of the items on the following list are your only motivation, I suggest you reconsider this choice.

Reasons Not to Become a Doctor:

- ✓ My parents are doctors
- ✓ The hardest thing I could think of doing
- ✓ I said I wanted to be a doctor and now I can't back out
- ✓ Everyone will respect me
- ✓ Someone said I couldn't do it
- ✓ I want to make a lot of money
- ✓ I have high grades, so I should probably go to medical school
- ✓ People expect it from me

Doc Talk

Money should not be a reason or a motivation for going into medicine. People who choose this profession for financial reasons will take our field in the wrong direction. As physicians, we need to remember that it is our primary goal to provide for our patients. If you focus too much on money, you might start to think that our patients are providing for us!

–Dr. Rickesh Sood, 2nd year family medicine resident

Just getting into medicine for prestige and money is not worth it. Because right now, in residency, there's no prestige and no money!

–Dr. Jennifer Graham, 1st year paediatrics resident

Do I Really Want to Be a Doctor?

I love my job. I can't imagine being as personally fulfilled doing anything else. As a lifestyle, though, medicine can be hard. The perception of what life as a doctor is like is often only loosely based on reality. Take some time to ask yourself these questions and think about your own motivation for applying to medical school. You only live once. Medical education takes a huge chunk of your time. Make sure it's really what you want to do.

Am I comfortable in emotionally intense situations? Do they make me feel more alive? Are they overwhelming?

Medicine is intense, and as a doctor, you'll be in the thick of it. Whether a patient is revealing that they're considering suicide, is worried about their child, or is in pain and afraid, the emotional intensity is high. Don't pretend that this is not going to affect you. If you're an empathic person (and I'm hoping you are if you're considering medicine), then you'll feel some of what your patients feel, and it can be draining. Other times, being part of this intensity can make you aware of the breadth of the human experience. How do you usually handle emotional intensity? Do you have mental strategies that allow you to process these types of experiences in a way that makes you stronger, or are you more likely to avoid these types of experiences and have them affect your ability to concentrate?

Am I a pleasure delayer?

A quality that you'll find in the majority of physicians is the ability to put off immediate rewards for greater rewards in the future. This type of personality seems to be able to work for hours, months, or even years without the possibility of gain in the near future. In medicine there are very few results that do not require significant personal investment, including the process of preparing for and applying to medical school.

What are my financial expectations?

It's true that there is a fair amount of financial security in becoming a doctor, regardless of what field of medicine you eventually choose. However, there's a lengthy time period between deciding to become a doctor and actually making the big bucks (over ten years if you decide during your undergraduate degree). During this time you'll likely amass over $150,000 in debt, so medicine is definitely not a "fast-track" to financial success. From time to time you may hear how much a doctor has earned in a given year, but medicine is a business, and this must be taken into consideration. Imagine a doctor who bills $300,000 in a year. Out of this money must be deducted the salaries of one or more clinic nurses, a secretary, rent and utilities, and medical supplies (cotton swabs, sheets, gloves, educational material, sterile trays, computers, examination tables, etc.). After subtracting the expenses from the $300,000, the remainder is cut in two, because you'll be in the highest tax bracket; the bracket where half of your income will be owed in taxes. Other doctors work in groups that share resources (such as staff and office space), but these doctors have to pay a certain amount of their billings to the organization or hospital. After all of this, you'll still be able to live comfortably. However, if you dream of super yachts, a second house in Europe, and your own horse ranch, this might not be the best route.

How important is sleep to me?

Preparing for medical school, getting through it, completing your residency, and actually being a doctor leaves few hours left in your day. Your sleep pattern is guaranteed to be thrown off during your training (medical school and residency), and likely will continue to be sporadic depending on the type of medicine you choose to practice. People who love an extremely organized sleeping and eating pattern might cringe at the idea of getting out of their perfect circadian rhythm. Certain areas of medicine are more forgiving and allow you to work more traditional hours, but this is a luxury that will have to wait until after your residency. Until that point, there will be years of sleep deprivation, regardless of what type of doctor you want to be.

This is an example of a week I've recently had:

Monday:
> 5:55 a.m. the alarm goes off
> 7:30 a.m. - 5:00 p.m. in the OR

Tuesday:
> 5:55 a.m. the alarm goes off
> 7:30 a.m. - 8:30 a.m. rounding
> 8:30 a.m. - 12:00 noon clinic
> 12:30 p.m. - 3:30 p.m. consults
> 3:30 p.m. - 5:00 p.m. reading

Wednesday:
> 5:55 a.m. the alarm goes off
> 7:30 a.m. - 2:00 p.m. consults in the ER
> 2:00 p.m. - 3:00 p.m. in the OR
> 3:00 p.m. - 5:00 p.m. consults on the floor
> 5:00 p.m. - 7:30 a.m. Thursday morning covering Labour and Delivery

Thursday:
> 7:30 a.m. - 8:30 a.m. Grand Rounds
> 8:30 a.m. - 9:30 a.m. rounding on my patients
> 9:30 a.m. - 2:30 p.m. home sleeping

Friday:
> 5:55 a.m. the alarm goes off
> 7:30 a.m. - 8:00 a.m. rounding on my patients
> 8:00 a.m. - 10:00 a.m. clinic patients
> 10:00 a.m. - 2:00 p.m. consults in ER
> 2:00 p.m. - 5:00 p.m. academic teaching

Saturday:
> 6:30 a.m. the alarm goes off
> 8:00 a.m. - 7:00 p.m. cover Labour and Delivery

Sunday
> Sleep in until 11:00am
> 7:00 p.m. - 7:30 a.m. Monday cover Labour and Delivery
> 7:30 a.m. - 9:00 a.m. rounding on my patients
> 9:00 a.m. go home to sleep

I'm very fortunate that I'm in a program that does twelve hour shifts on weekends instead of twenty-four, and I'm allowed to go home in the morning after I finish rounding on my patients— most programs make you stay until noon before you can go home.

How important is control over my own time?

When you're a medical student and a resident, you're a slave to the system. There will be a certain number of residents and at least one of you has to be available every hour of every day. A call schedule will be made up and you'll have to pull your weight. If you're sick when you're supposed to be on call, someone will have to fill in for you and you'll have to make the time up later to keep things fair. Often, you can request to not be on call certain days, but this is not always possible. You may discover there's a teaching session after hours, or a presentation you have to do, or you need to fill in for someone with little or no warning. It's sometimes difficult to make plans in advance as time off has to be booked and approved. When you're on call from home your pager may go off in the middle of dinner and you have to get up and head into the hospital. You'll work on holidays. You won't always make it home for Hanukkah. You might spend Christmas Eve in the hospital and have to leave your son's birthday party before he blows out the candles. Most people are open to trading shifts and honouring requests in the call schedule, but it can't always happen. Be prepared to miss something that's important to you at some time.

How do I feel about being constantly evaluated?

As a medical student and resident and as a physician you will be continually evaluated and re-evaluated on your performance. You will be quizzed daily and expected to be persistently adding to your knowledge base. The "brain break days", when you can just sit back and listen, are few and far between!

Am I easily frustrated?

What frustrates you? What do you do when you become frustrated? There are many aspects of being a doctor that are frustrating, and you need to be able to keep your cool, keep focused, and stay professional. It's frustrating to feel like you can't get something right. It's frustrating when you spend hours trying to educate patients who then choose not to follow your advice. It's frustrating to be operating and being unable to stop the bleeding. It's frustrating when you want to find a nursing home for a patient of yours and you cannot get them in because of an administrative technicality. If you're easily frustrated, you'll probably find medicine extremely stressful.

How do I feel about working for a long time with no guarantee of success?

The statement refers both to the process of applying to medical school and to the job of medicine itself. As stated before, it's difficult to get into medical school and there are many people who work towards it without being accepted. The application process is lengthy, and there's no formula to guarantee your success. In medicine, the same is true. You may work long and hard to treat someone, but there's no guarantee that they'll be helped. You need to be comfortable with this possibility.

How do I react to failure?

Many people need to apply more than once before they're accepted to medical school. Are you going to give up after one application, or will you take the time to learn from your past, find out what went wrong, and then do everything in your power to improve your chances next time? I promise you that at some time during medical school you'll feel like a failure. So mentally prepare yourself. This is hard, because many people who become doctors are used to being winners. They were top of the class. They'd won awards. They were the smart kid. Peers looked up to them. Now, those same people walk into the hospital and find themselves saying, "I don't know," more than they ever have in their life. You'll be embarrassed and humbled. You'll do things wrong. You'll not be able to answer the question when everyone is watching. This happens to everyone at some point or another, and it's hard. So how do you react to failing? Can you recognize other aspects of your life when you've failed? Can you take it and learn from it?

How do I react to the feeling of helplessness?

While becoming a doctor, you may feel awkward, amazed, thrilled, and terrified all in one day. At times you'll feel extremely helpless with a patient, while at the same time feeling a sense of duty towards them. In your early years, patients will often ask you questions you cannot answer. They'll want to know why can't you operate on this type of cancer or how long it will be before they will recover. Will their work allow them time off for their problems? Can you tell them exactly how much bleeding is normal? or can you predict if they will I be disabled? Even if you have your medical text books memorized, there's a lot you will not know until after you've been practicing clinical medicine for some time. Even when you've been practicing for many years there will be questions you can't answer and patients you can't help. Will you deal well with feelings of helplessness and newness?

Am I comfortable with people who have fundamentally different views from mine?

It's important to have a sense of self, a set of values on which you can draw to make decisions, and criteria that define right from wrong that help you act ethically and morally. But are you flexible enough to include views that are different from your own? Is one of your values a respect for differences, an understanding that two reasonable people can make different choices, and that what's right for you might not be right for someone else? Do you value a person's ability to make autonomous decisions on their own behalf, and would you protect and support this person's decision even if it differed from your own? People come to doctors for help and advice. Part of protecting your patient is honouring your patient's right to make their own choices regarding care—even if the choices they make are at odds with your expertise. This is part of providing compassionate, ethical care.

Is medicine something that will prevent me from being involved in certain things that are important to me?

What are you willing to give up and what do you hope to gain? Doctors do live rather hectic lives, but for some people this makes them feel more alive; they live on the constant challenge. There are many doctors that are married and are parents, and they require extraordinary time-management skills to feel involved with both work and family life. If you find that you are the type of person who is involved in multiple activities simultaneously, you will probably have to cut down on something in order to have enough time to study and care for your patients. You might not get away as much on holidays, and you'll be working weekends. However, there are some amazing opportunities for doctors to travel. Often, this will take you beyond the tourist tract, as you participate in medical care in underserved regions of the world and attend medical conferences overseas. There is a give and a take, and you need to decide if you're comfortable with the trade-off.

How do I feel around sick people?

Not all aspects of medicine are bloody or gory, but as a doctor in any field you'll be in intimate contact with people who are sick. Sick people have rashes, they have problems with their bowel movements, they bleed, they vomit, they cannot bathe as much as they would like to, they urinate accidentally. And they come to you, asking for help. You'll have to inspect and touch their wounds, put your fingers into orifices and sometimes cut into them. Are you able to treat these people with dignity? How would you react if someone vomited in front of you or told you they were in pain because of extreme constipation? Can you take care of that person with compassion without being embarrassed, condescending, or frustrated by their condition? Most people are turned off by blood, bad smells, and sickly looking people. Are you? Can you be truly empathetic and remain professional while helping them?

How do I see myself as a person in my 20's and 30's? How about in my 40's, 50's or later in life?

If you're applying to medical school in your twenties, you'll spend most of your twenties and possibly part of your thirties preparing to enter medical school, getting through medical school, and in residency working extreme hours. You'll probably spend your thirties establishing yourself in your career, finding a group or hospital at which you would like to work, and paying off the debt you acquired while in training. Some people suddenly discover that they've worked away their youth, or missed the opportunity to start a family while young. Their thinking had always been to accomplish some other task before they were ready to make any type of relationship commitment. Others successfully juggle the responsibilities of work, being a member of a family, and paying off their debt at the same time. Doctors are rarely unemployed, and often continue to work past the traditional retirement age. Some people choose to take on more academic positions that require less strenuous working hours later in life, whereas some still get up at three in the morning to go to the OR if they're needed. What do you see yourself doing at different stages of your life?

Am I comfortable with ambiguity?

Medicine is a science-based pursuit, and many people who apply to medicine are comfortable with "how things work" from this perspective. You will find, however, that although there is constant, active research in all fields of medicine, there are many more questions than answers. Not every decision you make will have a scientific backing, and you'll constantly have to remind yourself that medical research always pertains to a certain population of people, which may or may not represent the person you are treating at the time. On top of all this is the suitability of a particular course of action for a particular individual. You'll find there is also an art to this science, and different experts will come to different conclusions from the exact same problem. You'll also see the exact same condition in different people and see that they require different treatment for a variety of personal reasons. There are no set flow charts or algorithms in existence that fit each disease or patient uniformly, despite great efforts from medical textbooks at leading you to believe otherwise.

There are only guidelines, and you need to be comfortable moving within and through these guidelines based on a particular situation, and be comfortable with the constant debate of how to properly treat someone. You also need to be comfortable with the ambiguity of the constant evolution of medicine. As more is learned and discovered, these guidelines will evolve, and things that you thought you were doing right may prove later to be inadequate or even wrong. In the end, it just comes down to doing your best within current guidelines, and being willing to admit that in the future there may be better alternatives than there are today.

How do I envision the everyday lifestyle of a doctor, and on what am I basing this assumption?

Trust me— life in a hospital is not like being on ER or Grey's Anatomy. Medical students do not crack chests without supervision (they're lucky if they get to use a scalpel), tests take hours to come back, you don't have just one patient each day with a rare and wonderful medical illnesses to treat (a more realistic day includes twenty or thirty), and most doctors do not look fantastically coifed at 3:00 a.m.

You'll work very hard, sleep very little, and you'll carry the weight of your decisions and actions with you. That being said, you'll be part of an intimacy that few people experience. The glory is most often quiet - a sense of having noticed the right thing, a staff person saying "good job," or a patient's thanks. Most lives are saved not by risky and glamorous procedures, but by quietly and consistently paying attention, bravely asking questions, following up on your suspicions, making the right decision before things get out of hand, and not getting sloppy with the quality of care you provide. Emergencies do happen, but the majority of good doctoring is simply listening and preventing. If you want to know what the life of a doctor is like, find one and talk to them, shadow them, see how everyday medicine is preventative and unlike television leads you to believe...not very sexy. You'll save more lives taking routine blood pressures and talking about vegetables than you ever will performing CPR.

What sort of stability am I expecting?

Once you're admitted to medical school, chances are you're going to become a doctor. For many people, the stability associated with this job is very attractive, and although the job itself is stable, the job location, at least for the first six to ten years of your medical training, is anything but. Most people are not admitted to every medical school, and chances are that you'll have to move from one city to another in order to attend. During medical school, there are often mandatory rural placements that will take you away from city-based school for weeks and sometimes months at a time. Where you train for residency is determined by a process called "The Match," which I'll cover in more detail later, but many people are required to move again to a specific city with which they've been matched. During residency, many programs again have mandatory rotations that are in other cities. This entire process can be quite chaotic and somewhat unpleasant if you went into it expecting stability!

After you finish residency, you will need to find a job. Although there will be employment available to you somewhere, it may not be in the city you ultimately want to live. For example, if you do a cardiac surgery residency and want to return to your home town in rural Manitoba, you could face difficulties in finding employment. Such a small community hospital may not have the volume or the resources to require a cardiac surgeon.

Am I ready to go through puberty all over again?

The whole journey, from the initial dream of medicine, to the uncertainty of the application and the rollercoaster of highs and lows you'll experience on a daily basis is really like going through puberty all over again. There is a sense of constant growth that's both wonderful and exhausting. I know that my world view has changed since becoming a doctor, as I grew from a young and fresh medical student doing my first night of call (I was so excited about it I told the staff person, "Guess what! This is my first night on call EVER!"), to becoming a resident with multiple patients, learning obligations, as well as teaching assignments. You'll find few doctors who say they haven't felt overwhelmed or insecure at some point. The lows are balanced out by amazing highs—if you let them. If you're ready for this, then you may be ready for medicine.

What do I really want to get out of this anyway?

Go over your motivations, your dreams, and what you want from life. Do you feel this is the best way to lead a purposeful life? When you look back on your life when you're old and grey, do you imagine yourself satisfied with the life you've chosen? Do you really feel this is your choice, and not that of your parents, mentors, or spouse? If you're up for the adventure, if you feel a real sense of vocation, if you're aware of the personal sacrifices you'll have to make along the road to becoming a physician—if you're aware of all this and you still can't imagine doing anything else, this is the job for you.

Why Apply to a Canadian Medical School?

1) The number one reason to go to medical school in Canada is that it allows you to practice medicine in Canada. If you want to be a doctor in Canada, the most direct route is to go to medical school in Canada.

Currently, Canada is fairly strict about who they allow to be licensed as a doctor in this fine country. For the most part, to practice medicine in Canada, you have to have completed a residency in Canada. This is the 2-6 year training period following medical school graduation. Residency positions are allocated through CaRMS (Canadian Residency Matching Service), or the Match, which is a process not unlike applying to medical school all over again. Graduates from Canadian medical schools get the first chance to match to a residency spot during the first iteration of the match. Graduates from foreign medical schools are able to apply to the first iteration of the match in every province except for Saskatchewan and Alberta. However, although Newfoundland, Nova Scotia, Ontario, and British Columbia allow you to apply to the first iteration, you must apply to a "parallel" stream. This means you must apply to certain seats available only to international medical graduates, and this therefore limits your opportunities. These provinces also have a "return of service obligation" for international medical graduates, which could limit your mobility after finishing residency. Quebec and Manitoba do allow international medical graduates to compete directly with Canadian graduates for residency positions, and there are no return-of-service obligations. Therefore, although it's possible to get a residency position if you go to school abroad, your choices and mobility may be limited.

CaRMS: http://www.carms.ca

2) Lower tuition: It is less expensive to go to a Canadian medical school than a foreign medical school. Going to medical school abroad usually means that you'll be paying higher tuition, as the government'll not assist you. In Canada, medical school tuition is supplemented by provincial dollars, which you'll not qualify for otherwise. Cost of living is also sometimes higher overseas, and there is an increased travel cost each time you return home to visit.

3) More loans are available to you: Many provincial loan programs do not provide assistance at all or provide minimal assistance to Canadian students studying abroad. For this reason, you'll have higher expenses (as mentioned above) and lower available cash flow.

4) Social support: If you grew up in Canada, chances are that your family and friends are here too. Medical school is stressful, and knowing that your family and friends are closer to you (even if they're in another province) can make you feel less overwhelmed and can provide much needed support during stressful times.

A Canadian medical degree is very valuable. You can practice medicine in the United States with a Canadian medical degree without jumping through too many hoops, whereas practicing medicine in Canada with an American degree is more difficult. A Canadian medical degree gives you the versatility to practice medicine where you want in the future.

PART II:
GETTING IN

CHAPTER 4: DOCTOR DEVELOP THYSELF!

Extracurriculars and Social Development

"To the love of his profession the physician should add a love of humanity."
—*Hippocrates*

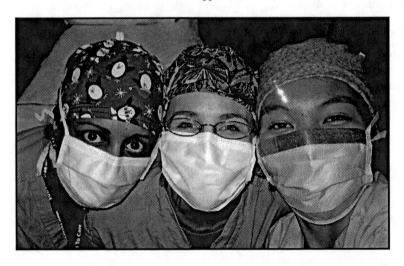

BECOMING a doctor starts years before you apply. Getting good grades in high school and university will make you technically eligible to apply, but development of yourself through interesting work and volunteer activities will give you the skills you need to succeed in medicine. Using your time to better yourself and your community will allow you to see if spending time with sick and vulnerable people is really for you. Although medicine can be difficult to "try before you buy," experiences that challenge your perceptions, your ability to communicate, and your ability work in an emotionally charged environment will help you know if you'd enjoy a career in medicine, and if medicine is right for you.

Doc Talk

It's been important for me to see the variety of personalities of people who are in medicine. There have been some people who don't seem personable outside the hospital but are really wonderful when you see them with patients. It's inspiring to me in that there is such a diversity of people who can work in medicine.

—*Midori Yamamoto, 4th year medical student*

I don't really know where the drive came from, I just knew it was something I wanted to do, and I can't imagine doing anything else.

—*Dr. Sandra de Montbrun, 3rd year general surgery resident*

I think you can never really know what medicine is like before you're in it. But you can never really know what anything is like before you're in it. So you have to have some really solid reasons to get into it, or you won't last. If it takes you a couple extra years to figure it out, go for it. That time is not wasted.

—*Dr. Jennifer Graham, 1st year paediatrics resident*

Medicine requires more then knowledge of science and a desire to help people. A physician has the multiple roles of medical expert, communicator, collaborator, manager, health advocate, scholar, and a professional (Canmed guidelines).

The capacity to excel at these roles is demonstrated by the following non-exhaustive list:

- ✓ self-directed learning
- ✓ time management
- ✓ leadership
- ✓ teamwork
- ✓ initiative

- ✓ creativity
- ✓ dedication
- ✓ communication
- ✓ an understanding of cultural determinants of health
- ✓ self-motivation
- ✓ commitment
- ✓ achievement
- ✓ problem-solving skills
- ✓ critical thinking
- ✓ scientific reasoning
- ✓ ability to listen and communicate effectively
- ✓ sensitivity to the needs of others
- ✓ adaptability and the ability to cope with stress
- ✓ ethical decision-making skill

You might have some innate ability in these areas already. If you do, you need to continue to develop them. If you don't have some of these skills but still feel that you want to consider medicine as a career, fear not! The ability to think critically, empathise, and listen can be learned and improved, just as your ability to understand Shakespeare or calculus can be improved through experience and practice. So how do you go about developing these less tangible but essential human skills? Through interacting with other people in a variety of contexts, and challenging your ability to communicate, to make decisions, to lead, to take initiative, and to listen. You need to have the opportunity to do things you've never done before. You need to be pushed to your limits and beyond. You need to be frustrated, afraid, angry, and you need to reflect on these challenges so you can grow and rise above them. As a physician, your greatest challenges will not necessarily be the intellectual decision of why a person is sick and how to treat them. You'll be challenged daily by questions you ask yourself: How can I develop a sense of trust with this patient? How can I truly understand his or her story? How can I better understand this patient's financial, social, and personality traits in order to plan proper care for them?

You'll need to make decisions based on sound ethical principles. Problems will need to be solved using a combination of creativity and scientific evidence. You'll be required to focus on a problem for an extended period of time without giving in to frustration or distraction. Your time must be used in a way that prevents you from being overwhelmed with the sheer volume of work that physicians face on a daily basis.

Personal growth can be achieved by participating in a number of activities outside the typical classroom environment. Many of these experiences can be categorised as follows:

- ✓ fine arts
- ✓ healthcare
- ✓ literature
- ✓ athletics
- ✓ organisation
- ✓ teaching
- ✓ travel
- ✓ working with under-serviced populations
- ✓ research

You're unique from everyone else who is applying, and you should try to find some activities within these categories that suit your individual personality and style. Not every doctor was that captain of his or her basketball team. Not everyone traveled to a developing country or served as the president of their student body. Most of those accepted have, however, participated in a diverse grouping of these areas with a high level of commitment.

Doc Talk

Part of doing extracurriculars was just getting to know my community. I joined a Japanese drumming ensemble, I was a rower for a dragon boat team. I also was volunteering at an epilepsy clinic.

–Midori Yamamoto, 4th year medical student

In my undergrad, I remember thinking I had to get into medical school, and I was thinking, "What does the admissions committee want?" and not necessarily "What do I want?" which is kind of sad. I wish I'd thought less of what the committee wanted and more about what I should have done to prepare on a personal level.

–Dr. Rickesh Sood, 2nd year family medicine resident

If you have a chance to participate in any healthcare activities or with an under-serviced population, take it. These opportunities can be found in many places and circumstances; in hospitals, doctors' offices, home-care environments, nursing homes, elementary schools, pregnancy centres, homes for the elderly or shut-ins, homeless shelters, isolated parts of the country – the list is endless.

It's essential that you find an opportunity to work with PEOPLE. The important part of this type of activity is that you can find out if you enjoy working with an "at-risk" population. This is also an excellent opportunity to develop your communication, empathy, and leadership skills while developing an appreciation for the multitude of factors that can contribute to the concept of health. If you're comfortable in this environment and feel you've done a good job, your supervisor would be in an excellent position to write a letter of recommendation for you when you apply to medical school. It's an added bonus if your supervisor happens to be a physician.

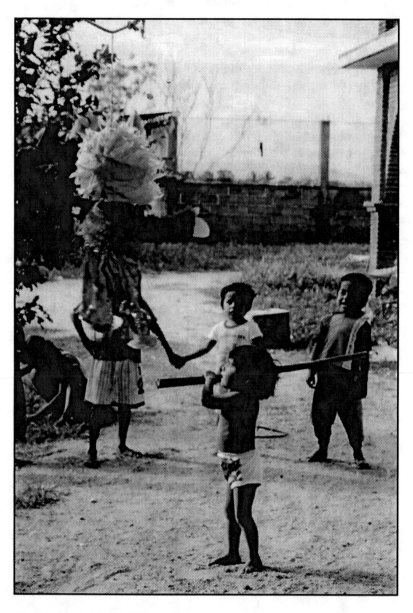

Children playing with a piñata in rural Mexico. I spent a summer during university in a cultural emersion program in Oaxaca and Guerrero.

Doc Talk

I actually went around the hospital, showed up in doctors' offices, and asked if there were any projects that I could work on with them. A lot of them said no, but a few of them said yes. I found some time to work with a home service group where I spent time with people with mental disabilities, and that was a really good experience because I got to work with them in their own environment. I got to see where they lived and what type of care they received, which I thought was really valuable. I also worked on some research in a biology lab. So after that I was able to say that I did understand what medical care is about. I worked for blood collection services, so I rounded on all the patients in the morning and I could observe what the residents were doing in the morning. I think I got good experience exploring both the social aspects of medicine and the research aspects of medicine. And because I was working with the pathologist I was able to talk to him about what doctors do. I decided that the next time I applied they couldn't say to me that I didn't know what a doctor did.

—Christopher McCrossin, 4th year medical student

You learn so much when you go overseas about how the world works.

—Dr. Jennifer Graham, 1st year paediatrics resident

The Cross-Cultural Experience and the Financial Factor

The Majority of doctors I know did, at some point, travel, work, or live in a cultural context that is different to the one they grew up in. This is probably in part a self-selecting group, in that people who are interested in cross-cultural experiences are also the type of people who want to become physicians. There's a concerning trend of fewer students from lower-socioeconomic standing applying to medical school. I don't know the specific reason for this; perhaps high tuition (*J. Kwong et al, CMAJ 2002;166(8)1023-8)*, more responsibilities at home and therefore less time available for academic and extracurricular pursuits, or less money available for organized activities. These are merely guesses. Regardless of your financial situation, if you want to have a cross-cultural experience there are ways of doing this without spending too much money.

1. Work with a cross-cultural group in your community. Volunteer with new immigrants to help them learn English or find their way around the city. You will have a great opportunity to learn much about where they've come from in return.

2. Go on exchange or host an exchange student while in high school. By living with someone's family and sharing your home in return, you'll have a more personal understanding of another country and culture. You may also learn a new language and potentially save money.

3. Have a cross-cultural adventure in Canada. Organize an exchange with someone living in Northern Manitoba, rural Quebec, a fishing village in Nova Scotia, or downtown Toronto.

4. If you want to travel abroad, see if you can work at the same time. Teaching English as a second language overseas is a classic way to teach and travel to many different countries. I know many people who have travelled to various countries including China, Vietnam, and Egypt. There are other programs available in Europe where you can get a visa that allows you to work for a specific period of time, usually six to twelve months.

5. If you decide to volunteer abroad, fundraise. Most programs that send volunteers abroad require you to pay for travel and living expenses. Have a garage sale, sell things on eBay, or hold a bake sale at your school. Solicit funds from various charitable organisations, and offer to do a presentation on your experience upon you return.

6. So develop yourself. Learn the skills you need to be a great doctor. Find organisations that are doing things that inspire you, or seek out needs in your community and start something yourself. This may take more time and effort, but you'll be participating in something meaningful to you and flexing your leadership, initiative, and creativity muscles!

Seek out needs in a community and start something!

- ✓ Meeting the need of senior home residents who lack recreational or social activities
- ✓ Walking neighbourhood kids home from school
- ✓ Cleaning or improving a local park
- ✓ Organizing or planning the restructure of an unsafe public area that is in need of attention
- ✓ Creating programs for shelter guests who are in need of life skills
- ✓ Guiding or touring new immigrants through your city or neighbourhood
- ✓ Starting an after-school soccer team for a local school
- ✓ Filling a need at a local Hospice
- ✓ Assisting people with disabilities on vacation

Look around you and you'll find opportunities waiting for you!

Doc Talk

When I was looking for a patient experience, I was initially assigned to help feed patients. I wasn't really enjoying it, and so I stopped. I then found that I could help with physio in the pool, and I felt like I was really getting to know people. When I was asked in my interview about the feeding assistance program, they knew that I didn't enjoy it. My advice to you is find a volunteer activity that you actually really like.

–Christopher McCrossin, 4th year medical student

I worked as a camp counselor at oncology camp. It was neat that is wasn't just for kids with cancer, but also for their healthy siblings and other family members. It was just like any other kids' camp, but with a little extra training at the beginning. Because it was a camp that attracted people who were interested in health in someway or another, it was a great environment to discuss things.

–Midori Yamamoto, 4th year medical student

In terms of volunteering, it was something my sisters had done a lot of, so I really looked up to them in that respect and decided that it was something that I wanted to do to.

I volunteered with the Red Cross starting when I was sixteen. I used to play a lot of community basketball so I ended up coaching with them and refereeing with them. I also volunteered at a retirement home; I would go once a week and do carpet bowling with the residents, which was really enjoyable. There was a resident who I used to spend a lot of time chatting with who didn't come one week, and I found out he'd passed away. I think that was the first time I thought about death and mortality. I think it really affected me. It was an important experience.

–Dr. Rickesh Sood, 2nd year family medicine resident

Choosing The Ideal University Courses

Really, when you're deciding what classes to take in university, I cannot stress enough that you need to take something that interests you. People really do get into medical school from a varying number of disciplines, including Applied Science, Arts, Computer Engineering, Teaching, Math, Midwifery, Music, Kinesiology, Nursing, Science, Law, and Pharmacy. (http://65.39.131.180/ContentPage.aspx?name=M.D._Prog_-_Admissions_-_Selection_Process)

Most medical schools have specific courses that you need to take before applying, but a few, such as Calgary, Western, McMaster, Northern Ontario, and Dalhousie require no specific courses prior to admission. The courses typically required are often first-year or second-year courses, so taking the prerequisites shouldn't keep you from pursuing the degree of your choice. Even if not a requirement, there is almost always an advantage to taking at least Biology, Physics, Chemistry, and Organic Chemistry, as they will prepare you for the MCAT, and when there are prerequisites, these often fulfill those requirements. Most medical schools also require English, humanities or social sciences courses, and statistics or biochemistry. If you haven't taken any of the above mentioned courses in your university years, there are two medical schools that do not require specified courses prior to entry, nor do they require the MCAT—McMaster and Northern Ontario.

Generally, I'd recommend that you take at least the courses that will prepare you for the MCAT, plus a social science. It will give you the greatest breadth of applications and give you a chance to test some of the material. Do you even *like* biology? Do social sciences interest you at all? Take the courses and find out. Have a look in the appendix for more details on course prerequisites.

Doc Talk

Because I started in an arts program, I had to take some catch-up courses during the summers.

—Midori Yamamoto, 4th year medical student

Taking organic chemistry was definitely something that I did solely for the committee and not out of interest. Even focusing a lot on the sciences in my undergrad was to get into medical school. I started to think, what the hell am I doing? Why am I taking courses I'm not interested in? I remember I was in advanced genetics because I thought I should be, but I hated it and ended up dropping the course. At first, my major was in biology, but I decided to double major and took social/cultural anthropology, which I loved. I did amazingly in it because I really enjoyed it. I wish I had done my entire major in anthropology and taken biology for how it related to anthropology. When I think about it, medicine is not that far away from a combination of biology and anthropology - bio is the science and anthro is the application to society and culture. And when you think back to that, it makes sense that I ended up in family medicine. I practice from a science perspective, but when providing primary care, I can be the person the patients really rely on. That can be really uplifting and a lot of fun.

—Dr. Rickesh Sood, 2nd year family medicine resident

We need more people with social sciences and arts backgrounds. It gives you a whole other way of thinking. In liberal arts, there is no right answer; there is only the best answer for the situation. Nothing is cut and dry. I think it really adds to medicine to have people from a variety of backgrounds with different experiences.
I did have to teach myself quite a bit when I was in medical school. I think that you should follow your heart, and do what you want to do, and later if you want to apply for medicine, go for it.

—Dr. Jennifer Graham, 1st year paediatrics resident

The GPA

Your GPA is one of the most important criteria when it comes to getting into medical school. Most schools use the GPA as the initial reason for rejection; if you do not have the required GPA, the rest of your application is not even considered. This is the most tangible and efficient way for medical schools to decrease the number of remaining applicants that need to be reviewed further. There are a number of ways that this first round of down-sizing is done: your GPA alone may fall below a fixed number, your GPA and your MCAT score may be combined and fall below a set figure, or perhaps only the top 50%, based on GPA alone make the cut-off (a figure which may change as the applicant pool changes). Regardless, when it comes to grades, higher is better.

When your GPA is being calculated, each school has a different system, so your admission GPA may vary from application to application. For example, School A might weigh your most recent grades higher than the ones you received in first year university. School B might weigh them all equally. School C might weigh your prerequisite courses such as biology, chemistry, and organic chemistry at 1.5 times the weight of all the others. Take the time to go through the admissions calculations carefully before you submit your GPA. You might find that you have a significantly higher GPA at school A than at School B, and you'll therefore have an increased chance of being accepted at School A.

In general, the GPA used for entry into medical school is based on your undergraduate grades. Graduate marks are often not looked at, even if you now have a PhD. You may get a few bonus points added to your GPA if you have a graduate degree, but it's the undergraduate grades that really count. It's essential that you maintain a full course-load during your undergrad degree, as this is often a requirement or at least a strong preference when applying to medical school. I've heard horror stories about students who spread out their courses over the summer so the load is lighter during the year, only to discover later that they're not eligible to apply to certain medical schools because they did not have a full course-load during the year. You need to be able to maintain your high grades while taking five courses simultaneously, not three or four. Not taking a full course-load doesn't necessary exclude you from applying to medical school completely, as some schools have different formulas for calculating GPAs when university was done part-time, or may require you to have a minimum number of years at full-time to be considered.

The pressure to maintain a high GPA during your undergrad can be quite intimidating, especially when you're transitioning to a new environment and maybe even a new city. Your course work is much heavier and less-directed than it was in high school, and getting A's suddenly requires more work than it used to. It's even harder if you're not certain if medicine is what you want to do and you want to explore in university. The transition from high school to university requires some fundamental changes, and these changes take many people their entire first year to figure out.

1) There's no homework.

Suddenly there's no one telling you to go home, study these pages, do these practice questions, prepare this for tomorrow. You'll have to be self-motivated. Read what the outline says, and stay on top of things by doing questions provided in your texts—without being told to do so.

2) The volume of work is at least three times that of a high school course.

The amount of work can feel like a punch in the teeth the first time you suddenly realise how much there is to do. You've been warned.

3) Go to tutorial.

They said it was optional, right? And isn't tutorial for people who don't understand what's going on? No, it's where essential things are taught! I'll admit to you that during my first year, I thought the very same thing about my calculus tutorial, until the day I realised the exam was based on questions gone over in that tutorial.

4) Remember that your marks count.

Years later, they'll still count. If you do poorly in these two years, it will be quite difficult to recover. Even if you're now doing a PhD in the subject you got a C in during your first year of university, the admission committee might look at your low mark in chemistry from seven years ago and it could be held against you. Again, each school is different, and some schools may allow you to drop certain courses if you've completed a significant number of other credits or years. There's a standard formula for grades at each institution, and for the most part, they're quite weighted towards undergrad performance. So, don't slack off!

5) University is filled with people who are just as smart and motivated as you are.

It's much easier to get A's in high school than it is in university, and this can come as quite a shock to many university students who were at the top of their high school class. In university, all your fellow students were once at the top of their high school class.

Doc Talk

After going through the process, I realised that my grades mattered a lot more than I thought they would. You often hear people say, "Do what you're interested in, it doesn't matter." I took on that philosophy, and took some courses that I had no aptitude in. Later on, I discovered that you can actually audit the course, so you can go through it for interest without being graded on it. I should have actually done that, so I could do it out of interest if I knew I wasn't going to do phenomenally in it. Looking back, if I'd done that it would have altered my GPA more favourably.

—Midori Yamamoto, 4th year medical student

It's important that you're in a program you enjoy because if you're happy you'll probably do better in it. You also need a program that either encompasses the prerequisites for medical school, or has them available as an elective. There are a number of courses that are prerequisites that contain material that you'll rarely use as an actual doctor. Sometimes, it really does seem that the courses are just there as extra hoops to jump through. I probably would have benefited more from taking a sociology, religion, or ethics course more than some of the courses that were required in my program. There are a couple of strategies that students use when choosing their courses:

1) GPA boosters:

Every school has a few courses that are just easier to get a high grade in than others. Often, they'll have material that you might be interested in from a more personal perspective, rather than an academic perspective. I took two courses that were fairly easy to get high marks in, for the most part because I'd already taken courses that covered some of the same material. I took a "Life in the Universe" course, which was a physics course that focused on astronomy, concluding on the factors that influence the probability that life will evolve. I learned a lot about red-shift, different types of stars, and the expansion of the universe, which was all fascinating. It was also pretty easy to understand because I'd already taken university level physics. Another course that was probably a GPA booster was an introduction to nutrition course. I'd already taken biochemistry at this point so it was a pretty straightforward course. Ask around - there's probably a course or two that is easy to do well in if you're motivated.

2) Taming your monster:

Organic chemistry was by far the hardest course I took as an undergrad, and many people will agree with me on this point. Organic chemistry does tend to pull down people's GPA. However, it's a course you need to take in order to properly prepare for the MCAT, and it's a prerequisite for certain medical schools. Some people choose to take this course during summer school, since certain schools do not count summer school grades in the calculated GPA. This way, you'll end up with the required course without having to report the grade. You also might do better in the subject if it's the only course you need to focus on during that period of time. If you're trying to maintain a full course-load at all times during the school year, it's important to remember to take an additional course from September to April in order to maintain your full coarse-load status. If you choose to pursue this path, it's a good idea to take a course you know you'll do well in, or a course with a light work load, rather than choosing a course from a year above you, one that requires extra time, or one that you might struggle to understand. This will protect you from inadvertently lowering your grade.

3) If there's a course that you're interested in but don't have any aptitude for, why not audit it? You'll get the exposure you want for your own interest, without it affecting your grades.

The Plan for Getting Good Grades

I don't think there's any magic formula, and things that may work for one person do not always work for another. I remember being told once that no one ever got into medical school without doing at least four hours of homework a night. So, in the hope that following this advice would lead to an acceptance letter, I spent a year heading out to the library each night at 6:00 p.m. Each night I would study diligently until the library closed. I would go faithfully to the fireplace room in the Stauffer Library at Queens University. I would sit in the chair and force myself to study—willing myself into medical school. I know that I watched an entire year of seasons go by through those long windows.

It didn't work. My final grades that year were just shy of what I wanted, and I knew that I would have to work even harder the next year to make them acceptable even with averaging them out.

The next year I had more freedom in my choice of courses, and I tailored my studying to the course. The classes with five hundred people and multiple-choice finals demanded that I memorize literally hundreds of cue cards that sat in towers on my desk. Most multiple-choice tests required you to recognize the correct answer, so that's what I would train myself to do. Other courses asked that you actually understand what was going on, so I would get old exams from the library and draw pictures in multicoloured markers showing the feedback loops and amplifications of hormones and transcription enzymes. For my undergrad anatomy exam, I realized that I had a real working model available during the written exam (myself!) and learned to flex and extend my muscles in sequence to help me remember. I was much more relaxed the following year. I'd study at the library between classes and be home at night. I enjoyed myself much more, and my grades went up significantly.

In general, if you're going for the grade, find out what you're actually being tested on and how. Cue cards can be good for memorizing large quantities of facts, and past exams are generally helpful for any test you're going to write. If you find that you're having difficulties, suck it up and get yourself a tutor. I got a tutor for Orgo and she really helped me scrape by.

Sometimes it's hard to stay motivated. Sometimes you'll wish that it was okay to just pass and take the pressure off. This can be especially hard when the idea and the dream of medical school seems so far away and abstract. When I was feeling really unmotivated and wishing it was okay to just have mediocre marks, I would take a break and do something completely unrelated. During exam time I would give myself an hour to eat and watch something on TV before resuming my studying. Sometimes I would read through medical school websites, which reminded me why I was doing all this work and motivated me to keep plugging away. It really is a long haul - an exercise in extreme pleasure-delaying. But I know I wouldn't be here now if I hadn't put in those hours, hadn't forced myself to review things just one more time, hadn't taken that one extra practice exam. The daily dedication and the sprint at exam time are worth it.

It's bizarre that a few marks here and there could mean the difference between being above or below the GPA cut-off. However, if you don't make that cut-off, the admissions committee will never know about you and will never invite you to an interview, and you'll never become a doctor. Just take it one step at a time, one exam at a time. Reward yourself if you're doing well. Take a step back and make a new plan if you aren't.

Recovering from a bad year is very difficult, but it is possible. If you're committed to medical school but do not have the grades to get in, you might consider taking an extra year of courses or even a second undergraduate degree. If you do well on these undergrad courses, it will dilute the poor grades you had previously. Some schools weigh your more recent marks more, or if you have enough years of undergrad grades, discount your early ones all together.

The MCAT

"Of all the hoops you have to jump through, the MCAT is the Hoop of Fire."
—*Dr. Sandra de Montbrun, 3rd Year General Surgery Resident*

The MCAT (Medical College Admission Test) is an all day long exam covering the topics of biology, chemistry, organic chemistry, physics, verbal reasoning, and a writing sample. The test is available twice a year in April and in August. Many people choose to write it after their second year of university because this is when they've completed the same material in school and it's fresh in their minds. I think of this as a "naked exam." You cannot bring in any type of aid, including calculators (and there's a fair degree of physics requiring math). Starting in 2007 or 2008 this test will be converted from a paper and pencil test to a computer-based test. You'll be provided with scrap paper, a pencil, and industrial-quality earplugs.

There are many different routes you can take to prepare for the MCAT. There are practice books filled with sample questions, practice tests available on the official web site, plus a multitude of commercial courses. I'm sure many people have prepared for the MCAT in a variety of ways, with varied degrees of success. Personally, I took the Kaplan course and found it quite helpful, mostly because it forced me to sit down and practice. It also gave me the opportunity to write mock exams in a testing-type environment, paying attention to the clock. Whatever you do, prepare. The MCAT is a long test and I suspect it takes more than just mastery of the material to make it through – it takes endurance.

Doc Talk

I borrowed the Kaplan test materials and I just studied the materials. I didn't take the course but I studied in the park for a month and a half. It was hard because I'd taken the previous year off.
I've heard of people saying that they prepare for [it] maybe just a week before, but I don't really believe that anyone really does that.
—Christopher McCrossin, 4th year medical student

I ended up registering for an MCAT course at the end of my second year, but I wasn't certain I would actually write it, so I sort of only half-studied for it. I just wanted to get to know what materials were available. I wanted to get familiar with the level of skill required, and I also got to know what other students were doing to prepare to go to medical school. I then actually wrote it at the end of my third year. I didn't retake the course. I just used all the materials. I wrote the August MCAT because my April university exams were at the same time.

—Midori Yamamoto, 4th year medical student

To prepare for it, I took the required courses, so I took chemistry, physics, organic chemistry, and biology. I took the summer before the August MCAT to study for it, and during that summer, I took Kaplan. I chatted with people who'd taken it, listened to the horror stories, and visited the AMCAS website to look at the practice questions on there. They give you one a day, but they're exhausted in about forty days. I definitely prepared. The course helped because I was forced to sit down and focus. It was also good because I had to drive downtown to take the courses, and that required a certain commitment since I was in an isolated environment. I could have taken Princeton, but it was where I was going to school and it would have been with people I know. It might not have been as conducive to studying.

–Dr. Rickesh Sood, 2nd year family medicine resident

Registration for the MCAT takes place in early January for the April exam, and in early May for the August exam. You need to register online at http://www.aamc.org/mcat. The cost of the exam is US$210 dollars at the time of the printing of this book. If you fail to register in time, the late fee is US$50. If you've written the MCAT three times already and you want to write it again, you need to provide the AAMC with proof of your intent to apply to medical school.

The MCAT, as stated before, is a full-day test. You write for a total of 5 and 3/4 hours, with a one-hour lunch break in the middle. The schedule is as follows:

Physical Sciences - 77 questions in 100 minutes
10 minute break
Verbal Reasoning - 60 questions in 85 minutes
Lunch - 1 hour
Writing Sample - 2 questions in 60 minutes
10 minute break
Biological Sciences - 77 questions in 100 minutes

The Physical Sciences Section consists of multiple-choice questions covering physics and non-organic chemistry. You'll be required to know conversions between imperial and metric measurements (this is an American exam so it's still littered with feet, yards, quarts, and pounds). You'll also need to have an understanding of physics at a first-year university level, and an understanding of non-organic chemistry. Your math skills have to be reasonably strong, as you're often required to perform functions such as logs without the use of a calculator. Many answers are rounded and therefore do not require an exact answer, just the most correct. University courses that prepare you for this section of the MCAT are first-year general chemistry, first-year physics, and a first-year calculus or similar math course.

The Verbal Reasoning Section is again made of multiple-choice questions, this time from social sciences, humanities, and natural sciences. You're not required to have prior knowledge of these subject areas in order to answer the questions; you're being tested purely on your ability to comprehend and analyse the passage presented. The topics can be as diverse as Victorian Dress, the social implications of city planning, or the history of a musical instrument. Courses in subjects that force you to read critically such as history, politics, and English may help prepare you for this section, but there's no specific course selection needed as long as you've developed some skill in analytical reading.

Lunch is the easiest section of the MCAT, as long as you remember to actually eat something healthy (not a good time for indigestion), have something to drink to keep yourself hydrated, and use the bathroom.

The Writing Sample does not require any previous knowledge to complete. You'll be given a statement and then usually asked to prove and then disprove it, followed by resolving the conflict. For example, the statement might be "Winners are made, not born." You must first explain the statement (e.g., Winners are people who succeed, and success comes from hard work. Therefore, winners are made and not born). You must then provide an example of when the statement is not true (e.g., Sometimes there are disciplines, such as Olympic-level track-and-field, that require a massive amount of natural talent and ability to stand a chance of becoming a winner). You must then resolve the two statements (e.g., generally, winning and success comes from hard work. However, there are situations at the extremes of competition, when only those with the correct set of natural abilities are able to be winners).

You can find a list of practice writing-sample statements here:

http://www.aamc.org/students/mcat/about/wsitems.htm

Taking a course that requires essay writing at a university level may help to prepare you for this section, but as with the verbal reasoning section, there's no specific course selection as long as you have the writing skills needed for this task.

The Biological Sciences Section covers material from first-year biology and organic chemistry. This section requires a basic understanding of genetics, embryology, cell biology, physiology, and principles of organic chemistry. Taking a first-year course in biology and taking organic chemistry (often offered as a second-year course) will have you generally well prepared for this section.

MCAT Scores Explained

Verbal reasoning, physical sciences, and biological sciences scores are converted from a raw score to a number from 1-15. The number you receive corresponds to a percentile score, with 15 being in the highest percentile and 1 being in the lowest. In this way, you're really being scored against all the other people who are writing the MCAT, so if it was a particularly hard or easy MCAT that year, the people who did the best will still have the highest score and can compete fairly with those who wrote it at a different sitting. Most medical schools consider MCAT scores above 9. These numeric scores are sometimes added together from each section to give a total MCAT score, e.g., 28 or 31.

The writing sample is given a letter score from J to T. Each of the two writing samples is given a score out of 6 by two different people. These scores are all added together to give you a final numeric score that's converted to the letter score. This means that if you do really well on one essay and poorly on the second, you would get the same score as if you did moderately well on both.

I researched this section using the official MCAT website, which can be found at: http://www.aamc.org/students/mcat/start.htm

MCAT Timing Strategies

April vs. August MCAT

1) Writing the April MCAT during your second year of undergrad

This option gives you the maximum number of chances to write the MCAT, whether you're applying to medical school in your third or fourth year, and you'll know your score before you send in your application.

If you do poorly on the MCAT, you can re-write it in August and still apply during your third year.

The other advantage is that you'll likely have just finished covering the material that's on the MCAT in your university courses such as biology, chemistry, and physics, so you may be more mentally tuned in to the MCAT.

However, university final exams are usually written in April as well. Your grades are very important to keep you application competitive, and it could be difficult to divide your study time between your university exam preparation and MCAT preparation simultaneously. I've heard of students writing the MCAT on the weekend and then an organic chemistry exam on Monday. Just the thought of that makes me exhausted! Many people also choose to take a prep course before the MCAT; if you chose to do this you might have conflicts with your current university classes and exams.

2) Writing the MCAT in August between your second and third year

You have the benefits of just finishing the pertinent course work without the stress of studying for and writing your university final exams at the same time. It might be easier to attend an MCAT prep course during the summer months when your schedule may be more flexible.

In my opinion, this is the optimal time to write the MCAT if you plan on applying during your fourth year, since you'll have recently covered the material featured in the MCAT. Taking the MCAT at this time will also allow you to see your MCAT mark before you send in your application. You can then divide the work of applying to medical school between two summers, using the first summer to prepare for and write the MCAT, and the second to prepare your package and request and obtain letters of recommendation.

3) Writing the MCAT in April of your third year

This could be an awkward time to write the MCAT, because up to a year may have lapsed since you studied the material. You'll also be preparing for exams on different topics, and you might find it difficult to take a pre course on another topic. However, if you're applying to medical school during your fourth year, it does give time to re-write the MCAT if you do poorly the first time.

4) Writing the MCAT in August between your third and fourth years

It will have been a year since you took the core preparatory courses for the MCAT, but at least you won't be trying to study for exams and the MCAT at the same time.

You will have an opportunity to take a prep course, but you'll also be working on your applications at the same time.

If you're not attending a university, then the best time to write the MCAT is when you have the time to study and prepare adequately prior to the exam. Obviously, this will not be the same for everyone depending on their personal situations.

The Importance of the MCAT

The importance of the MCAT depends on your school of choice. McMaster, Ottawa, and the Northern Ontario School of Medicine don't even consider the MCAT when choosing applicants, whereas some schools only use it as a flag if the score is quite low. Other schools use it as the deciding factor when determining which applicants should be interviewed. Having a low score will not necessarily get your application tossed out completely (particularly if it's in one particular section), nor will a high MCAT score guarantee you admission to the school of your dreams. Most MCAT admission averages hover around 10, which is a solid mark. So study, do well, and get over this hurdle to get to the interview. Look in the appendix for specifics on minimum and average MCAT scores.

The day before the MCAT, I did the following:

1. Didn't study (at this point, there's nothing more to learn).

2. Drove out to my test site and found the room so I wouldn't be late looking for room 4A2300 the next day.

3. Made a lunch plus snacks and drinks and put it in the fridge (can't rely on cafeteria food).

4. Laid out my clothes for the next day (I have these very comfortable stretchy pants with dragons on them) and brought an extra sweater just in case.

5. Packed a bag with pencils, my MCAT registration package, and my ID (even with all that they will fingerprint you when you enter the room).

6. Watched a funny movie

7. Set my alarm clock so I could show up half an hour before registration if the traffic was an hour longer than my practice drive (nothing makes people panic like being late for something important).

8. Went to bed early to get enough sleep but not so early that I couldn't fall asleep.

Day of the exam:

1. Got up with alarm - DO NOT HIT SNOOZE (set a second alarm clock across the room, or have someone else to check to make sure you're up if you have a history of failing to wake

on time).

2. Took a shower to wake up.

3. Put on dragon pants.

4. Ate breakfast.

5. Double-checked contents of bag, took my lunch out of the refrigerator.

6. Drove to test site.

7. Wrote first half of the exam.

8. Ate lunch outside, enjoyed the sunshine and did not allow myself to be caught up in the conversations of either "Oh, that was way too easy," or "Well, at least I can write it again if I fail."

9. Wrote second half of the MCAT.

10. Went to red lobster, put on a bib, and ordered the lobster feast.

Try, Try Again

You can write the MCAT three times, after which you need to get special permission from the AAMC to write a fourth time. If you did poorly on the MCAT, you still have options. If you notice that your test is not going well on the actual day of the exam, you have the choice to void it up until the last section is finished. If you void your exam, it will not be seen by anyone, and your score will not count. However, because you wrote the test you cannot get a refund for it, and it will count as one of the three permissible tries. As discussed before, writing the April MCAT gives you the opportunity to take it again in August if you're not happy with your score. If you know where your weakness lies, then you can tailor your studying around that area. Generally, your MCAT scores are valid for five years. Different schools use re-written MCAT scores in different ways. Some take your best score, some your most recent, and some average them. You should call each school directly regarding their MCAT policy.

CHAPTER 5: THE APPLICATION

Inside Your Application Package

START early and organize yourself. This is a lengthy process that requires running around, contacting people, and coming up with a brilliant way to present yourself. You need to start your preparation the summer before your planned year of entry. This will ensure that you get your official transcripts sent out in time. This approach will also allow enough time for the AMCC to send your MCAT scores to the correct schools and for the people giving you recommendations to organize their letters.

Application package checklist:

1. Calculated GPA for each school you're applying to.

2. Write to AAMC to forward MCAT scores to appropriate schools if not already done.

3. Contact each school you attended as a university student and have official transcripts sent to each medical school.

4. Contact potential reference letter writers, provide them with a copy of your CV, ask if they want a meeting, and give them a pre-addressed envelope.

5. Write CV.

6. Contact people who can verify each statement on your CV and ask permission to use them as a verifier.

7. Write a personal statement for each medical school you're applying to, if required. Make sure it's in the required format and length, and answers any specific questions.

The application package is generally made up of your GPA, MCAT scores, a personal profile that contains a list of extracurricular activities, research work, leadership experience, athletics, a personal statement, and letters of recommendation. It's this package that determines whether or not you'll be invited for an interview.

GPA: This is something you've been working on steadily throughout your undergraduate years. Some schools calculate your GPA as a straight average throughout your years at university, while others weigh later years or certain courses more heavily than others. This is, for many schools, the first cut-off point. If you do not have the required GPA, the rest of your package will generally not be considered.

MCAT Scores: The MCAT is also often used as an initial cut-off score, and is required for all schools except Ottawa and the Northern Ontario Medical School. McMaster considers the verbal reasoning section of the MCAT only.

Personal Profile: Many schools require a CV or a personal profile. On the OMSAS (Ontario Medical School application Service) application you express everything you've done with your time since age sixteen. Other applications look at the time spent since you started university. Make sure you have the name and contact information for someone who can verify each of your extracurricular activities, and contact them before you send in your application. This way, they're aware that they may be called to discuss your involvement. I sent emails asking if it was all right to use them as a contact person, and requested a phone number they were comfortable having listed on my application package.

Writing Your Personal Statement

This is your first opportunity to let the application committee know who you really are and why you're suited to medicine. Some people start this statement with a quote or experience that they feel summarizes who they are or what drives them. I think the key to a good personal statement is to make it *personal.* The letter should sound like it came from *you* instead of a generic statement, and should show that you're an interesting and diverse person. If it's filled with clichés and broad statements, it will be void of character and there will be nothing to distinguish you from every other applicant.

You'll probably be writing a number of personal statements at the same time. Try writing a base letter first, and then tailor each letter to each school. Before I started writing my personal statements, I went though the extracurricular and volunteer activities, and tried to think of an experience that illustrated each of the concepts that needed to be addressed in my letter. I also tried to find experiences that illustrate who I am, what drives me, and why I thought I was well-suited for medicine. This is very personal, but after reflecting on your motivations, it will be easier to express why you want to become a doctor.

The reason why you want to organize your experiences and think about specific incidents and learning moments, is because a statement is always more believable and carries more weight if it can be substantiated by an actual event. As an example, compare these two statements:

Statement 1:

"I feel that health is determined in part by culture, because a person's perspective of their illness affects how they feel and interact with other members of the community."

Statement 2:

"During my summer in Tonga, I learned that women are expected to start having children in their early twenties. I saw a woman who was thirty-two and expecting her first child. On her chart it said, "geriatric pregnancy." The cultural norms of Tongan society dictated that this was an unusual event, while in North America it is very common for women to have their first pregnancy in their thirties. Her culture saw her as unhealthy, and while I was speaking to her it was evident that she was embarrassed to be so old! It was this experience that taught me about the power of culture as a major determinant of the experience of health."

The second statement makes the same point as the first, but is reinforced when linked with a real experience, making it appear more genuine, and lets the reader know that you not only understand your statement, but that you understand how it applies to real life.

Another example:

Statement 1:

"When I'm not achieving my potential in a particular area, I can be counted on to work harder. The drive to improve myself continually is one of the traits that makes me suited for medicine."

Statement 2:

When I was the ancient age of twelve I decided to learn to dance. Most girls start ballet training when they're four or five years old, but I wanted to learn anyway. When I was dropped off for my ballet class in my pink tights for the first time, I looked around and saw that it was filled with girls half my age. The music started, and although I did my best to keep up, I had a burning sense of humiliation building up inside me. I was awkward. I was too old to be there. I was going through puberty and wearing spandex in public. I would be lying if I didn't tell you that I cried that night. As horrified as I was to be put in the beginner class, I realized that I had to make a decision. Was I going to return the next week, or not? I decided that if I really wanted to learn to dance, I was just going to have to keep showing up and working harder than everyone else. So I donned my pink tights and returned the next week. Within two years I was in a dance class with people my own age, and I continued dancing and performing right through university. This experience taught me that I can make the decision to push myself, to work through what seems like an impossible task, and achieve a goal.

Doc Talk

On the application, they ask a lot of specific questions, and it's easy to answer in sort of a naive way. I think they're looking for something a little more concrete. As opposed to saying, "I want to help people," give an example of how you want to spend your day.

—Chris McCrossin, 4th year medical student

Even if you don't plan on applying until your fourth year of university, if you have the prerequisites I think it's a good idea to ghost apply during your third year. Apply even if you don't think you'll get in, because it's really helpful to go through the application process once.

—Dr. Rickesh Sood, 2nd year family medicine resident

I had some friends in psychology who were helpful with the wording of my application.

—Dr. Jennifer Graham, 1st year paediatrics resident

Big Mistakes to Avoid

1. Addressing the wrong school: e.g., "I'm excited to be applying to the University of Toronto Medical School because…" written on an application to the University of Ottawa.

2. Spelling errors: This makes it look like you're sloppy with your work.

3. Bragging or putting other people down: No one wants to work with someone who comes off as arrogant or who does not appreciate other members of a team.

4. Lying: Just don't do it. Not only is it behaviour unbecoming of a future doctor, but if caught, it may prevent you from applying to medical school for an extended number of years

5. Not answering the questions: Many medical school personal letters ask that you answer specific questions in your letter. Not answering the question or skimming over it makes it seem that you didn't read the directions. Would you want your doctor to skip over reading the directions?

6. When asked if you have any faults or failures, stating that you have none except that you work too hard: Sorry, get real. There's

no way that any human being can make it though twenty or more years of life without doing at least something that you regret and learned from. If asked this question, dig deep, be honest, and write about something that you were actually responsible for (as opposed to a failure from your environment). Make sure you include the learning experience that went with the regret.

For example, stating that your greatest failure was, "Not finding a research position for the summer because I was studying such a prestigious area of science that there was no one to work with," sounds like you're blaming others for not knowing as much as you. It also gives the impression that you're not taking responsibility for the fact that you could not find a position. It would be better stated, "I was extremely interested in a very particular area of science, and I made the mistake of not even considering other areas of research. As the summer approached, I realized that not only had I failed to find a position researching my area of interest, but there were no research positions left in any area. I ended up working at a movie theatre that summer, which I'd done during high school. I learned that by being stubborn and overly particular, I ended up loosing out on other opportunities. The next year, I started early, and considered a wide range of options for the summer. I actually ended up teaching English in Korea for four months. My failure to expand my horizons that first summer, followed by the amazing culturally different environment of Korea last summer, taught me the value of flexibility."

As a medical student, you'll be facing ethical, intellectual, and social challenges everyday. You need to be able to assess yourself honestly and continually work toward being a better doctor. Give the persons reviewing your application the opportunity to see that you possess this ability.

Getting Letters of Recommendation

Usually, two to three letters of recommendation are needed for each medical school application. Always give your referees one or two months notice before you need to submit their letter. Ask for a letter in a way that gives them a chance to say no if the letter is not going to be excellent. For example, you could say, "I'm applying to medical school, and I was wondering if you felt that you knew me well enough to write a strong letter of recommendation?" Provide the referee with a copy of your resume. If you've worked with the referee, provide them with a list of specific initiatives you've taken. Offer to meet with them to discuss the letter. If you've seen a copy of the letter, its weight is lessened. Give your referee a pre-paid, pre-addressed currier envelope so all they have to do is place the letter in the envelope and send it. Make sure it's as little work as possible for them.

Who Should Write your Letters of Recommendation?

The people you choose to write your reference letters should know you extremely well and be able to make comments on your character, personal qualities, and academic capabilities. Make sure that all of these aspects are covered, but they need not be all in the same letter. For example, your boss from when you were a camp councillor at diabetes camp can comment on your character and personal qualities, and the person who supervised your undergraduate thesis can comment on your academic capabilities and work ethic. Usually at least one referee should be a non-academic or character referee. You may feel that a well-known or high-profile referee will increase your chances of getting in. However, I would think that a detailed letter from a less-famous person is worth more than a generic letter from a high-profile person.

Personally, I got letters of recommendation from my boss at the Ontario Science Centre (I'd worked as a host there for a number of summers), from a home for children with disabilities where I'd worked, and from a physician who's lab I'd worked in for two summers. I felt this was a good way to show the different facets of my personality. The letter from the Science Centre showed my ability to teach, take initiative, and interact with people. The letter from the home for children with disabilities showed that I had experience and the ability to work with people who had special medical and social needs. The letter from the physician showed that I had the intellectual capacity and curiosity to be a doctor.

Many people I know were accepted into medical school had a letter of recommendation written by an M.D. But how do you go about getting to know a doctor well enough for them to write a letter for you?

1. Do an honours degree or 4th year thesis. You'll have the opportunity to have small classes and get to know your professors. If you're taking human biology courses you may have an M.D. as a professor who'll be able to get to know you. By doing a 4th year thesis, you may have the opportunity to work with an M.D. or PhD as your supervisor. You'll have the opportunity to get to know them, and they'll be able to honestly evaluate your work ethic and research skills.

2. Find someone who knows a doctor. If you have a friend or relative in healthcare, maybe they know a doctor who is approachable and interested in mentoring. Many doctors often have small projects on the go that you might be able to help with.

3. Look through university department websites in anatomy, physiology, microbiology, epidemiology, pharmacology, etc. There are often profiles of the staff that work in these departments. See if you can contact an M.D. who is associated with the research and offer to volunteer in the lab.

4. Volunteer at a hospital in an area that requires a lot of interaction with people, for example, the Child Life department. See if you can meet with a doctor who's also involved with the same patient population, e.g., Paediatrics or Psychiatry, to get to know them. Ask them if there's any way you can have an expanded role in your volunteering.

5. If you're already a healthcare professional, there's probably a doctor you've worked with who you feel appreciates the quality of your work. They may be a very good person to write a letter of recommendation.

6. If you volunteer or work at a camp who is associated with a physician (these would usually be camps for kids with specific health concerns) you may get to know them over the course of the camp, especially if you make the effort to get involved.

7. Talk to your family doctor if you have a good relationship with them. They, or another member of their group, may be interested

in having some help around the office. Remember, any type of exposure is good, even if you're just showing patients to the room or helping with paperwork. I wouldn't ask a family doctor to write a letter of recommendation for me if she or he only knew me as a patient.

8. If you get the chance to work in or volunteer at a hospital, find out about grand rounds and see if you can go. It shows enthusiasm, and gives you a taste of the types of issues doctors deal with. If you get to know a particular doctor well enough through your time at the hospital, see if you can go to the departmental rounds. These are smaller and often less formal. Sometimes other members of the healthcare team such as nurses, researchers, and dieticians are invited. Not only does this show how keen you are, but it also shows you how healthcare teams use their problem-solving skills.

Doc Talk

I was working in a lab between undergrad and applying to med school and I got a letter of recommendation from my supervisor who was a physician. I also worked on an honours project during my fourth year, and I got an academic letter from my professor - he was also a physician. My third letter was from my music teacher. I thought it would bring perspective to my application to be recommended by someone who knew me through my teens.

—Midori Yamamoto, 4th year medical student

My letters of recommendation came from the director of a fly-in recreational program in the Northwest Territories that I used to work at. I went to Trent, a small university, so one of my prof[essor]s knew me quite well and was able to write me a letter. A physician that I met in Laos also wrote a letter for me.

—Dr. Jennifer Graham, 1st year paediatrics resident

Should I See My Letter of Recommendation?

Some application forms ask the referee if the student has seen the letter of recommendation, and it's possible that they carry less weight if you do. It would be more prudent to discuss what's in the letter without actually seeing it if you're offered to take a look. If you have a chance to get a copy of it after the interviews, it could be a good resource if you need a letter of recommendation at some point in the future.

CHAPTER 6: THE INTERVIEW

Preparing for the Interview

S O you've written a stellar application and that juicy package finally arrived in the mail. Now it's time for the interview. This is your opportunity to let them know what you have to offer. Your probability of getting into medical school has also just increased significantly! Congratulations!

To be adequately prepared for the interview you need to know yourself and your motivations for applying to medical school, and then practice, practice, practice.

Preparing for the interview is similar to preparing your application package. One difference, though, is that you don't know what questions will be asked during the interview. To combat this, you must ensure that you're comfortable with what you've gained from your past experiences, and that you're prepared to use your ethical decision-making skills. Anything that you write on your application is fair game, and it's not uncommon for an interviewer to pick a line from your CV and say, "Tell me what you learned, liked best, disliked, or wished you had changed about this experience."

See if you can think about an experience that illustrates the following phrases:

✓ self-directed learning
✓ time management
✓ leadership
✓ teamwork
✓ initiative

✓ creativity
✓ dedication
✓ communication
✓ cultural determinants of health
✓ self-motivation
✓ working with under-serviced populations
✓ commitment
✓ achievement
✓ problem solving
✓ critical thinking
✓ scientific reasoning
✓ ability to communicate effectively
✓ sensitivity to the needs of others
✓ adaptability and the ability to cope with stress
✓ advocacy
✓ healthcare
✓ literature
✓ organisation
✓ teaching
✓ travel

Writing them down can help you organize your thoughts. Go to the website of each school and see if there seems to be a theme at that school, such as research, primary care, self-directed learning, evidence-based medicine, or rural and under-serviced populations. Be prepared to answer questions about this topic and provide examples from your life that demonstrate your understanding in these areas. If you have an opinion about something, see if you can back it up with a real-life experience of yours that illustrates how you came to have this opinion.

Make sure you can answer the question, "Why do you want to be a doctor?" When you think about it, it's a simple but loaded question. If you're to become a doctor, you'll be spending the next six to ten years earning little or no money, studying extremely hard, staying up for thirty hours straight, and dealing with emotionally, intellectually, and physically exhausting problems. You should have an excellent answer prepared for occasions when interviewers ask you why you want to submit yourself to these circumstances in order to become a doctor.

Think about this one, and write it down. Saying you like science and want to help people is not enough. Talk to people who know you well. If you're switching from another career, think about why you're giving up what you've already established for yourself to start over. There are many lists of questions out there that people may ask you during an interview. Take the time to go over them and write a few sentences in response to each. Pay particular attention to questions you find challenging. You'll be glad you did in future interviews when you're able to respond with clarity and poise.

Doc Talk

The advice that a medical student gave me was to think of things in "black and white." If they ask you something, state a pro and a con. You want to identify things that you want to work on, and show that you have done something to try to improve it.

—Christopher McCrossin, 4th year medical student

Practice, Practice, Practice!

You need to become comfortable speaking about yourself without sounding like you have a canned answer for everything. Personally, I went to the career services office at my university to conduct a practice interview in front of friends. You can provide them with a list of questions, or ask them to make them up on the fly. The key here is to practice staying focused, organized, and enthusiastic. If you're especially concerned about speaking spontaneously, there are programs such as Toast Masters that give people an opportunity to practice speaking in public. There is a list of practice interview questions available to you in the appendix of this book.

Doc Talk

I practiced for the interview by having a medical student ask me questions and give me feedback. It was sort of embarrassing, but they gave me a lot of good feedback.

—Chris McCrossin, 4th year medical student

Be Positive!

Remember that although the interview is officially maybe two hours in length, the entire day counts. Be nice to the other interviewees; people (including those who make big decisions) will find out if you're jerky, name-dropping, or putting down other applicants. Think positive thoughts and try not to think of the other applicants as your opponents, as this will only increase your stress levels. Instead, try to imagine the other applicants as your future classmates and colleagues, which indeed they are.

The year that SARS hit Toronto and the surrounding areas, medical school interviews were suddenly interrupted. Hundreds of potential interviewees had to be re-routed out of the hospital to another building to uphold the lock-down. Everything had to be reorganized in a matter of days. A classmate of mine who was heavily involved in running the interviews donned an orange vest to help direct confused interviewees. One car pulled up, and when told they had to park elsewhere, the student shrilly said, "Do you realise who I am? I have a *medical school* interview and you're going to make me late! I have to park here!" The irate medical student in the car clearly thought the colleague of mine was a lowly parking attendant, and not a member of the admissions committee.

The moral of the story: treat everyone nicely. Everyone is as stressed as you are, so try to be your best and most polite self the whole day, regardless to whom you're speaking.

Doc Talk

There are eyes everywhere. You never know who you're talking to. The thing is, if you're a genuinely nice person you'll be fine, because you're generally nice and polite anyway. You want people who are genuinely nice in medical school. What if your patient comes in and they're unemployed? How are you going to treat them?

–*Dr. Sandra DeMontbrun, 3rd year general surgery resident*

The Standard Interview vs. the Multiple Mini-Interview

Currently, most schools in Canada have what is known as the standard approach to the medical school interview. This varies from school to school, but typically involves a single candidate (you) sitting with a small group of interviewers. The interviewers will ask you a variety of questions about your background your motivations and test your ethical decision-making skills. Based on your answers, the interviewers will decide if you'd make a good medical student and ultimately, a good doctor. If you go to a mock interview provided by career services at your university, most likely it will be of this type. However, the University of Calgary, the University of Saskatchewan, McMaster University, the Northern Ontario Medical School, and the University of Manitoba (alongside a traditional interview) all make use of a different type of interview; the multiple mini-interview, or MMI.

This is a new type of interview based on the medical OSCE (objective structured clinical examination), a type of exam used to evaluate medical students and medical residents. During an OSCE you rotate through a variety of stations, each with a standardised patient with a different medical problem. OSCE's are designed to evaluate both cognitive and non-cognitive skills such as communication skills.

The MMI, like an OSCE, requires the participant to rotate through a number of stations, each with a different examiner and question or situation, lasting about ten minutes. These questions and situations are supposed to test ethical decision-making skills, communication skills, collaborative abilities, critical thinking, and knowledge of the healthcare system. You're generally given a written prompt, asking a question or describing a situation, given two minutes to read and think about the prompt, and are then given eight minutes to respond to the question or act out the scenario. It's possible that you'll be asked to interact with an actor while the interviewer observes. Although most stations ask you to discuss a situation or scenario, standard interview questions may also be used.

Because you're evaluated by many different people, if you feel you don't get along with someone, that single opinion may be diluted.

You're also more fairly evaluated in comparison to your peers in that everyone has exactly the same questions to answer. If you perform terribly at one station you can start the next station afresh, without that interviewer knowing you had difficulties on the last one. By comparison, in a standard interview it might be harder to recover from completely fumbling a question. However, I highly recommend that you go to the library and get a copy of "An Admissions OSCE: the multiple mini-interview" *Medical Education* 2004:38:314-326.

In terms of getting sample questions for the MMI, they're definitely hard to come by. Medical schools using the MMI often ask the participants to sign a confidentiality agreement regarding the content of the interviews. However, I highly recommend that you go to the library and get a copy of *An Admissions OSCE: the multiple mini-interview Medical Education* 2004:38:314-326, which is the initial paper discussing the use of the MMI. In the appendix of this paper are ten sample questions for the MMI. These situations include the ethics of using placebos and the ethics surrounding circumcision, a passage that the interviewee is supposed to critically evaluate, and a few examples of communication skills situations. Get a friend and practice doing these examples in real-time - that's two minutes to collect your thoughts followed by eight minutes of interviewing or acting out the given scenario. I would also recommend that you find and read "The Ability of the Multiple Mini-Interview to Predict Pre-Clerkship Performance in Medical School" *Acad Med.* 2004 Oct; 79 (10 Suppl) :S40-2. I used both of these articles to research and write this section on the MMI. I would also recommend reading the fact sheet on the MMI provided by the University of Calgary at: http://files.myweb.med.ucalgary.ca/files/62/files/unprotected/MMI _FAQ.pdf

One Time at Band Camp: Real Life Experiences During Interviews

There will be a multitude of questions you'll be asked when writing your application, and again when interviewing. In my opinion, it's nice to have thoughts and feelings about things, but having actually acted in a certain way or experienced something gives you more credibility than stating how you feel or what you would do. Don't just state how you'd go about solving a conflict with a colleague. Give a real example of a time you were in conflict with someone and how you dealt with it.

Spend time soul-searching (when preparing for my medical school and residency applications I would often come up with examples when riding a bus or sitting in the tub), read your old diary, think about times in your life that changed who you are as a person. Look over your CV and think about a significant event, learning experience, or change that happened during each experience. Write things down if it helps you organize your thoughts, or brain-storm.

Remember, medical training will expose you to emotionally and physically strenuous experiences. You have to show that you're a person who's dynamic and willing to learn from your mistakes. Being able to reflect upon your life in such a way shows growth and maturity.

Think of a real life example of the following statements:

- ✓ Best job I ever had
- ✓ Experience or interaction with a healthcare issue
- ✓ Self-directed or independent learning
- ✓ Time management
- ✓ Overcoming a significant challenge
- ✓ Change of attitude
- ✓ Truth telling and integrity
- ✓ Resolving a conflict
- ✓ Making a mistake and what you learned
- ✓ Example of problem-based and experiential learning
- ✓ Creativity
- ✓ Leadership
- ✓ Research
- ✓ Human interaction
- ✓ Thinking clearly in an emergency
- ✓ Hard work
- ✓ Biggest failure
- ✓ Greatest success
- ✓ Advocate
- ✓ First experience that made you think about medicine
- ✓ Challenge
- ✓ Appreciation for complex systems or multidimensional problems

✓ Your understanding of biopsychosocial medicine
✓ When were you a teacher? A learner? Both at the same time?
✓ Confrontation
✓ Disappointed in yourself
✓ Helping people

Doc Talk

If they ask you, "Why do you think you would be a good physician?" say that you're good at something and then give an example instead of just saying I'm very caring or very honest, or I'm interested in the sciences. Tell them you're interested because of a project you worked on. Don't just say adjectives, link them to an experience.

—Christopher McCrossin, 4th year medical student

I did not feel prepared at my interviews; it was sort of on the fly. They were both very friendly interviews, not interrogative at all, more conversational. But they were so conversational that I didn't formulate them into, "This is why I want to be a doctor, this is why I want to do medicine," and so I think I didn't convey that message. Make sure that what you say during the interview, you tie it into why you want to be a doctor. There were some comments that caught me off guard. And then after the interview, of course I thought of an answer. When I was talking about my interests, I didn't tie it into my interest in medicine. One of my interviewers said to me during the interview, "You know, you should be a teacher!" That really took me off guard and I didn't know how to respond. It felt like an insult because I was here to interview for medicine. But of course, in medicine, there's so much teaching going on, you teach pretty much everyone you meet, and in medicine, it's such an important ability to have. But I wasn't thinking along those lines. I thought they didn't want me in med school and I should
go to teachers' college instead.

—Midori Yamamoto, 4th year medical student

I remember the first interview I had I was really uncomfortable. I was in a strange city, and I didn't really know what to expect. I was really comfortable at Mac because I really wanted to be there.

—Dr. Rickesh Sood, 2nd year family medicine resident

I looked up behavioral interview questions on the Internet and then I practiced with people. I thought of examples of what I did wrong and what I learned from it. There was a physician and a student who were interviewing me, and the student sort of drifted off. As soon as I finished answering a question, the student started paying attention again and asked me exactly the same question again, "Tell me a situation where you embarrassed yourself." So I had to scramble and come up with a second answer on the spot; I'd only prepared one response.

–Dr. Jennifer Graham, 1st year paediatrics resident

Ethics

I am including ethics in the interview section of this book because it's probably the first time you'll be formally asked about an ethical situation. You need to know how to approach it in such a way that demonstrates an understanding of ethical principles.

Ethics, for the most part, is actually quite logical, but it requires that you're able to understand the multiple factors that play into an ethical dilemma. My number one suggestion to better understand medical ethics and prepare yourself for the interview is to read *Doing Right* by Philip C. Hebert. It's a thorough review of a number of classical ethical dilemmas in medicine, and provides an approach to ethical situations.

As a doctor, you'll be required to act ethically every day. Personally, I consider ethical decision-making, like many aspects of medicine, both an art and a science. It's based on logical principles and an appreciation for the social, emotional, cultural, and personal events that shape people and their decisions.

You'll be faced with ethical dilemmas where there doesn't appear to be a right answer. In these situations you'll need to make a decision that's the lesser of two evils, does the least harm, and allows you to sleep at night. The decisions you'll be faced with will be complicated by time, resources, fears, your previous experiences, the amount of backup you have, information from higher-ranking staff, and your ability to make clinical judgments. There's often a lot of information to be taken into account and multiple people, perspectives, and values to consider.

Your resources and time are not unlimited and each decision you make as a physician affects not only the patient you're treating, but also the patients you're not treating. You can't be in two places at once, and any time you spend with one patient is at the expense of another. In the same vein, there's only a finite number of CT scans that can be performed in a hospital each day, only a finite number of hours available in the OR, and only a finite financial budget that must not be exceeded.

At times, you may be asked by more senior colleagues to do things that you're uncomfortable with. What would you do if, as a medical student, a doctor introduces you as a colleague to a patient? What would you do if you're asked to perform a vaginal exam on an unconscious patient who's undergoing neck surgery, because you need "the learning experience." How do you treat the pain of a patient who is recovering from a major surgery when your senior resident says, "Don't give him too much, he's just a drug seeker"?

You may have patients or families asking you for help in earnest, but your hands are tied ethically and legally. I was once involved with a palliative care team where a family was watching a woman die of COPD. She was gasping for breath, and although we were treating her pain and breathlessness as best as we could, her daughter cried out, "Please, do something! We treat animals better than this." It was a tragic and painful moment.

I've been with a man with a dementing illness living in a nursing home who was asking to be vaccinated for the flu like the rest of his peers. He'd been deemed incompetent and his wife, who is his executive decision-maker, tells us she does not want him to be vaccinated, as she feels vaccinations are dangerous. The geriatrician and I had to decide if we should vaccinate him or not.

I've worked with a patient who was thirty-three weeks pregnant and had a longstanding history of opiod use for a well-documented chronic pain disorder that was escalating during pregnancy. She was requesting stronger and stronger types of opiods and was demonstrating addictive characteristics. It was known that the opiod use was harmful to her baby. It was a challenge to find an ethical balance between treating chronic pain, preventing a more deeply entrenched addiction, and minimising exposure to her fetus.

A clinical clerk I was working with had a patient who switched back and forth with regards to whether or not she wanted resuscitation when she was in a deadly heart rhythm. She had already once declined at the last minute when the team was standing and ready to use electricity to reset her heart. She was again feeling palpitations and questioning if she wanted the treatment or not, and it appeared that maybe she did not understand what the treatment really entailed. The staff said she had previously made the decision against resuscitation and said that she was not to receive treatment. We had to decide what to do.

My male ob-gyn colleagues have been put in the situation where a woman in labour states that she only wants other women present during the delivery. It's a challenge to balance the wishes of the patient with the availability of female residents. The question is then often brought up - what if she said she only wanted a white person to deliver her baby? How should we act ethically then?

Ethical Questions During the Interview

Many interviews make use of ethical questions to learn more about your ability to work through an ethical situation, to see if you have an appreciation for the different sides of an ethical dilemma, and to learn more about your moral integrity.

You may be asked an open-ended question such as, "How do you feel about affirmative action?" You may be given a certain situation such as, "What would you do if a twelve year-old girl was requesting a prescription for birth control?" There are many tough questions to ask yourself in these types of medical dilemmas. Do you have an understanding of why this is a dilemma? Do you understand the pros and cons of the issue? Do you understand the points-of-view of all parties involved? Do you appreciate that there are immediate and long-term consequences? Is it okay to sacrifice one good for another? Is the autonomy of one person in conflict with the safety (or beneficence) of others? Is something being done for the beneficence of one person while justice is not being done for others?

State your thinking process aloud when you are answering the question. Remember, these are dilemmas, so there really is no single right answer. It's the process that you go through that's most important, so demonstrate your ability to think through a complex ethical situation. If you're asked to draw a conclusion about something ("what would you do?" instead of "what are the issues surrounding?") make a decision and be prepared to defend it based on ethical principles. This is easier to do if you begin by stating your understanding of the essential conflict and the colliding principles, rather than immediately stating what you would do.

It would be prudent to read around a number of "hot topics" in medicine and healthcare prior to your interview so that you understand the ethical issues surrounding them. The key is to appreciate both sides of the story. What complicates these issues?

Here's a short list to get you started:

✓ Abortion
✓ Euthanasia
✓ Spanking children/corporal punishment of children
✓ Censorship
✓ Futile treatment
✓ Privacy
✓ Public vs. private healthcare
✓ Reproductive technologies
✓ Sexual education of youth
✓ Legalization of marijuana
✓ Cloning
✓ Gene patenting
✓ Physicians attending drug-sponsored events
✓ Use of placebo effect
✓ Direct to consumer advertising
✓ Wrongful life
✓ Surrogacy
✓ You suspect a well-respected colleague or superior is acting unethically

Doc Talk

I was asked, "A man and woman come for fertility counselling. You find out that the man has no sperm. They come to you later for their results and the woman is pregnant. You have the two tests in front of you - the positive pregnancy test and the negative sperm test. What do you do?"

—Chris McCrossin, 4th year medical student

I was asked what I would do if someone in the group is not contributing to group work. Or what I would do if I was writing an exam and I see one of my colleagues cheating.
At some point you'll be asked the classic scenario: what would you do if you're scrubbing in on a surgery and you smell alcohol on the breath of the staff surgeon?

—Dr. Sandra DeMontbrun, 3rd year general surgery resident

I was asked, "What would you do if someone came in and refused to vaccinate his child?"
I was also asked, "A man is in your office and you find out he is HIV positive. He doesn't want you to tell his wife. What do you do?"

—Dr. Jennifer Graham, 1st year paediatrics resident

I'd also recommend paying attention to any recent news stories surrounding ethics in medicine. Be prepared to talk about a personal ethical dilemma and how you resolved it. Make sure that it's actually a dilemma, meaning that there was a conflict of principles that had to be resolved. Show respect for the importance of the principles and how you ultimately chose to resolve it. These types of situations often evolve while working in a group or on a committee, but you also may have been put in a situation where you had to make a decision like this on your own. It would also be important to reflect on times when you regretted how you handled an ethical situation.

The key points to take home from this are:

1) Understand that as a physician you'll be required to approach problems of an ethical nature on a daily basis. In fact, ethical considerations will be integral to your everyday activities. If you

want to be a doctor, you should be skilled at and enjoy this type
of problem solving.

2) The interview is an opportunity for the committee to evaluate
your capacity to work through ethical questions in a fair and
logical manner. It's your opportunity to show that you have an
approach to ethical dilemmas that takes into account certain
important principles, and that you're aware of some of the
important ethical questions in medicine.

Doc Talk

The classic question is about a Jehovah's Witness who is refusing a
transfusion. They want to see that you have a viewpoint on it and can
stand up to it. They may challenge you repeatedly by asking, "So are
you really going to let this person die?" You need to show that you're
solid in what you say, so don't flip-flop back-and-forth. Being
indecisive and not believing in your values are signs of weakness. You
need to understand the consequences of your decision, and stand by
it.

–Dr. Sandra DeMonthrun, 3rd year general surgery resident

When you're answering an ethical question, it's not the answer that's
important, but the thought process that you go through. It's okay to
say that it's a hard question to answer. Just talk through it. You can
come to a conclusion and say that in reality you would discuss this
with your colleagues. I mean, that's what medicine is all about.
Multiple minds looking at a problem.

–Christopher McCrossin, 4th year medical student

Interview Day Attire

Now, I'm not pretending to be an expert at this, but this is some
simple advice for going through the process.

1. You need a suit. It has to fit. It has to be clean and ironed. A
cheaper suit that fits is better than an expensive suit that doesn't.
If you're borrowing the suit (many people do) make sure you try

it on a few times before the interview so you don't have that first-time-in-a-suit look.

2. Most people wear dark colours. I've seen some cream-coloured and light-grey suits on interview day, but most people go for black, brown, or navy. You want the interviewers to be imagining you as a doctor and as a professional, so you need to dress like one.

3. Don't wear anything that could be mistakenly interpreted as sexy. If you're short, get a tall friend to stand near you to see if they can look down your blouse. You want your pants to glide past your bum, not wrap around it. If you're wearing a skirt, sit down in front of a mirror with your legs crossed and make sure you aren't showing any under-roos. Wear a bra the same colour as your skin to ensure it doesn't show through your shirt. Men should wear a tie and a dress shirt that isn't transparent or tight. An undershirt, if worn, shouldn't be seen through a dress shirt.

4. Be comfortable. Don't wear shoes that are new or shoes that will cause blisters. I think the best advice I can give you is to wear a jacket. You'll be sweating during this interview, don't kid yourself, and the thick material of a dark jacket will hide your soaking pits marvellously. Undo the buttons on it when you sit down to prevent wrinkling and pulling on the buttons, and do it up when you stand up to acquire that smooth professional look. Don't take it off. Wear your hair so that it will not fall in your eyes. Accomplish this without distracting hair ornaments.

5. Although you're dressing conservatively, you might want to add a bit of personality to your suit so you feel like yourself. A bright blouse or dress shirt, or a small, interesting piece of jewellery can add a subtle bit of personality.

6. Don't wear perfume or cologne, or heavily scented products. Not only are they distracting, but many hospitals actually have policies against their use.

7. Brush your teeth in the morning. Bring gum with you to chew after you eat any food. Spit it out before you go on any tour, have an interview, or speak with anyone. This is purely functional gum.

8. If you need one, get a hair cut a few days before the interview. Go for a tried-and-true look as opposed to anything that might make you feel self-conscious.

9. Piercings: People have differing opinions on this one. Some say that because you're interviewing to be a medical professional you should look professional, and therefore have no facial piercings. They do not want to be pre-judged on their potential to be a doctor. Others have said, "If they don't accept that I can be a professional and be who I am then I don't want to go there anyway." If you chose to keep more than your earrings in, keep it low-key. You want everyone to be focused on what you're saying and how you interact with people, not trying to figure out if your eyebrow ring is real or not.

CHAPTER 7: THE BACKUP PLAN

Henry Ford once said, "Failure is only the opportunity to begin again more intelligently."

WHAT do you do when your application does not result in an interview, or an interview does not result in an admission? Not everyone gets into medical school the first time around. So, you need a backup plan. In fact, you should be working on your backup plan and your medical school admission simultaneously. Many people need to apply to medical school more than once before they get in, and they make just as good doctors as those who got in on the first try.

Ultimately, if you're serious about becoming a doctor, you should be intending to apply again. It's important that you use the time between cycles to the best of your advantage. See if you can get feedback from the schools you applied to as to why your application or interview did not result in an offer of admission. If you attended the interview and felt there were questions you were unprepared for, write them down so you're better prepared for next year. Use this time to examine your application and look for areas you may need to improve in. Meet with an academic advisor at your university and go over your application, finding out if there's an area that you can improve in. Perhaps you need more experiences related to health care, or need to re-write the MCAT. You should be working on your backup plan concurrently with your application to medical school so you're not left hanging.

Doc Talk

After I didn't get in the first time, I gave it a month, and then I went in to speak to the dean of admissions to ask where I went wrong. I didn't get any concrete answers, but he did say that medically-related experience is important. You need to demonstrate that medicine is what you want to do. It was frustrating because they say you need medically-related experience, and at first when you try to get it, they say you have to be a med student. It's like the chicken and the egg. I eventually spoke with a pathologist who had coordinated one of the courses I took as an undergrad, and I got to shadow him. It was easier to get around the issues of patient confidentiality working with a pathologist. So that was a good experience. I shadowed a couple of the pathology residents, and that gave me a better idea of what doctors do. So the next time I interviewed and they asked me how I know what a doctor does, I had great answer for them. In my first interview they asked, "How do you know what a doctor does, and how can you really understand what you're getting into?"

—Christopher McCrossin, 4th year medical student

I didn't have a backup plan. Honestly, I think I would have just figured it out if it happened. I was just lucky.

—Midori Yamamoto, 4th year medical student

My backup was to go to law school. I'd already been accepted so I felt very comfortable about my future. I knew I didn't want to do pharmacy as a backup, and I didn't want to do dentistry because I have this thing with teeth. I didn't think I had the patience for teaching. I have a hard time with large groups of kids.

—Dr. Rickesh Sood, 2nd year family medicine resident

There are several options available to you should your initial plan fail. These options focus on improving your credentials while you continue to explore medicine as a career. This is not an exhaustive list, and I'm sure that those of you who are creative can find other useful ways to spend your time between application cycles.

Find out what went wrong and fix it

This is a very direct approach. Find out where your application is lacking and do something specifically about it. This requires you to anticipate where your application may be lacking before you find out whether or not you've been accepted. It means you can plan out volunteer work or school activities that could increase your chances. Remember that accurate self-evaluation is an excellent quality in a medical student, and you should be able to anticipate and plan around any problem. It's also very helpful if there's a policy of letting failed applicants know what they need to do to improve their chances.

If you're applying near the end of your third year of undergraduate studies, apply again toward the end of your fourth year

This option may appear obvious, but it gives you a real chance to improve your grades, continue working on your extracurricular activities, and perhaps re-write the MCAT. If fact, you'll now be quite experienced in the application process, so this time you'll be better prepared. It's important to remember that medical schools receive the applications in the fall, well before any final marks from the current year are available. So if you know this will be your backup plan should you fail to get in during your third year application, it's extremely important to keep your marks up during third year, because it will be your third-year marks that the application committee will see if you apply in your fourth year. If you're in a program that has a fourth year thesis option, take it. You may then have the opportunity to work with an M.D. doing research, which will improve your application and may lead to a great reference letter. You also will have another summer to fill with adventures, volunteering, and lab work. You really can improve your application over a one-year period.

Masters Degree, or if you have one, a PhD

This is a popular choice for people applying out of university. Most university students who are applying to medical school enjoy their course work, and are good enough at it to continue their education at a higher level. Graduate school gives you a chance to show your ability to do research and allows you to spend your time independently while making a small amount of money. Graduate students often have the opportunity to teach, travel, and present at conferences, all of which are feathers in your hat when applying to medical school. If you can, try to work with an M.D. You may get the opportunity to participate in some clinical aspects of research, find out more about being a doctor, and end up with a reference letter from a physician. Many medical schools will add a few extra points to your GPA if you have a master's degree or PhD. Be advised, though, some schools will not accept your application if you're in the middle of your program without a letter of release from your supervisor. So taking a master's degree may cause you to wait two years before you're able to apply again, but your application could potentially be much stronger. You should call the schools and read their policies carefully to see which require a letter of release or a completed master's degree.

Other Health Care or Helping Careers

There are many careers that allow you to use your brains to help others. Many of these involve patient contact, such as respiratory therapy or nursing. You may find that one of these careers actually suits you more than medicine does. By applying to one of these professional programs, you

1. Get a chance to increase your grades

2. Get exposure to patients and the healthcare environment

3. Develop interpersonal skills that will be valued if you decide to reapply to medical school

4. May be interacting with physicians, which will help you to better understand their role

5. May discover that you would rather be a physiotherapist, dietician, clinical geneticist, or occupational therapist, and are now graduating with a fantastic professional degree!

There are other professional programs that use many of the same skills as physicians that focus on helping others, such as interpersonal skills and logic and reasoning. These careers include law, public health, social work, and teaching. These should also be considered.

Check the appendix at the back of this book for listings of other healthcare careers.

Working

You may have the opportunity to work in an interesting environment that allows you to stay financially afloat and also helps you work towards reapplying. Working during the day gives you the opportunity to study at night if you plan to rewrite the MCAT, and the weekends are available if you want to do volunteer work. Work that involves research or interacting with people, especially in a healthcare setting, can be quite valuable. You also may consider working abroad, such as teaching English overseas.

Travel

If you're one of those lucky individuals who are able to pick up and go for a year, this might be the year to do it. If you do not need to improve your grades or rewrite the MCAT, you can find a number of interesting opportunities abroad. Even if you need to improve your grades, perhaps you can start out your adventure by taking a credit abroad. If you're serious about reapplying, there are a number of volunteer and work opportunities that can help develop your leadership and empathy skills, while increasing your understanding of the cultural determinants of health. Plan carefully, and not only will you have a year that you'll never forget, but you'll also become a better applicant and ultimately a better doctor in the long run.

International Schools

There are many medical schools internationally that accept Canadian students. England, Ireland, Australia, and the United States accept Canadians, as do a number of medical schools based in the Caribbean. Starting in 2007, Canadian citizens and permanent residents are eligible to apply to the first iteration of the Match. This is dependent on the applicant having never undertaken postgraduate training in the US or Canada, and applicants must also have passed the MCCQE. More about the specifics of this are available in the CaRMS section of this book. It's important to learn about your eligibility for a residency position in Canada following medical school abroad, because you usually need to have completed a Canadian residency program to practice in Canada. Applications can be expensive, and if you're applying to Canadian schools at the same time, be advised that international schools may want a deposit upon your acceptance. However, applying to both gives you the best chance of becoming a doctor. It is important to note that if you apply to and accept an international medical school spot, you can still reapply to Canadian schools during your first year abroad. For example, let's say you're accepted into a five-year medical program in Ireland. During your first year of Irish medical school, you reapply to Canadian schools and fly home for the interview. If you get the Canadian spot, you can withdraw from the Irish program and start your first year of Canadian medical school. If you are not accepted, you return to Ireland and continue medical school there. Either way, you end up with a medical degree, and with the possibility of completing it in Canada, which is less expensive and often takes less time.

Doc Talk

There was a guy a year ahead of me. His nickname was "Lucky" because he got the last spot. He got four interviews, was waitlisted, and got a spot two days before class started. He's now a family physician.

—Dr. Rickesh Sood, 2nd year family medicine resident

CHAPTER 8: YOUR STAGE IN THE GAME

I WANT to highlight some of the groups of people that might have special concerns or questions when applying to medical school. All of the previous information still applies, but hopefully you can take away something specific for yourself!

For High School Students

Your life as a high school student matters!

Goals to complete in high school:

1. Participate in extracurricular activities that help you develop and grow as a person, help you discover who you are, and diversify your interests

2. Prepare yourself academically for success in university by taking the courses you need and getting high grades

3. Chose a university that suits your personality and learning style

Let's start at the beginning; it's a very good place to start - The Sound of Music

If you're picking up this book during your high school years, good for you. Planning for a career in medicine often starts in high school. In fact, half of those who enter medical school decided they wanted to be a doctor either before or during high school. (2004 National Physician Survey: Medical Student Questionnaire.) Maybe you had an experience where you had a chance to be in charge at a critical moment, or perhaps you found yourself loving the dissections in biology class. Maybe you were intrigued by the way doctors are getting involved on a global level through projects like Doctors Without Borders, or advocating on behalf of countries devastated by the AIDS crisis. Maybe you heard about a new scientific breakthrough made by a physician, or maybe you're the type of person that friends go to when they need someone to talk to. Any of these experiences might make you consider becoming a doctor.

While in high school, many of your choices change the academic opportunities available to you in the future, and because you're in the process of discovering who your best self is, your experiences will affect the intrapersonal, communication, and empathy skills you have as an adult. As an adolescent, your brain is undergoing amazing and phenomenal changes, and the choices you make today will help to create the adult you'll be tomorrow. It's by choosing to challenge your leadership, communication, listening, and empathy skills that you can actually become a skilled communicator, leader, and listener.

I encourage you not to pad your resume. It's a waste of an adolescence. Resume padding is also fairly obvious and will only get you so far. Find things to do that you're sincerely interested in, whether you're good at them or not. Get out there and do something—make some mistakes and then try again. If you already have excellent intrapersonal skills, you're off to a great start, but you still need to push yourself and continue to grow.

Trying something new or hard will never be a waste. Even if you decide later on that you don't want to be a doctor, the people-skills you'll develop by challenging yourself and reflecting on it will serve you well in business, law, teaching, trades, and in your personal life. This is a win-win situation.

Experiences in high school can set you up for opportunities later in life. I feel that I was able to become a doctor in part because of how I spent my high school years. I participated in a number of sports such as swimming, cross-country, and downhill skiing. I tutored, took dance classes after school, and joined a number of clubs. I spent a summer in Oxford studying English. I applied to the Ontario Science Centre School, a program that takes students from across Ontario to earn senior science credits. My success as an applicant was probably a combination of my grades and extracurricular activities. I probably did well on the interview because I was comfortable presenting myself, a skill I'd developed by participating on the debate team and improvisation team (a competitive drama team that does sketches similar to those on "Who's Line is it Anyway"). Being a student at the Science Centre set me up for a summer job as a host at the Science Centre, which challenged my communication skills daily. One of my bosses from the Science Centre wrote me a letter of recommendation for medical school, and while interviewing for medical school, I was able to recount stories from working at the Science Centre to illustrate my ability to communicate in difficult situations. Let high school be your starting point.

Academics

People who become doctors tend to have good marks as high school students. High academic achievements in high school can open doors by qualifying you for scholarships, awards, special programs, and extracurricular activities. You're more likely to be accepted to the university and program of your choice, and you're more likely to be recommended for academic opportunities. If you plan to apply to medical school in the future, you should be getting mostly A's at the advanced level. In terms of courses, you need to make sure that you have the high school credits needed to apply to the university of your choice, and take the specified prerequisite courses. You'll need to have at least an advanced credit in Grade 12 English, biology, chemistry, physics, and calculus. However, different universities may have different prerequisite courses, so check with your guidance counsellor to plan out your course schedule.

If you have an opportunity to take a credit in an enriched environment, take it. Not only is the coursework a lot more fun, but you'll probably become more deeply involved with the material, resulting in a better understanding overall. Personally, I took my OAC English credit in Oxford over the summer, and took biology, physics and Science in Society as credits at the Ontario Science Centre. Here are some examples of ways you can get high school credit for things outside a traditional classroom:

✓ Take a language course such as French or Spanish in a country where it's natively spoken, or study French in Quebec or another French-Canadian community

✓ Take a history or English credit in a culturally relevant location

✓ Apply to the Ontario Science Centre School

✓ Find out about Co-op programs in your high school, and see what credits you can get for it. This would be especially valuable if you could participate in a healthcare field, such as doing ambulance ride-alongs, or working in a lab. If you're very fortunate there might be a physician willing to take a high school student on as a co-op student

✓ See if you can design a credit for yourself. I was eligible for a social sciences credit in high school for doing one hundred hours of tutoring and writing a final paper on learning abilities

✓ Find out if your school offers an outdoor education class. This is a physical education credit that involves trip-planning, camping, hiking, and canoeing skills. If your school does not offer this credit, approach a teacher or the principal about starting one

✓ Go on exchange. Most schools have some sort of exchange program. This is a relatively inexpensive way to travel, become comfortable in a second or third language, and expand your view of the world while receiving high school credits

✓ Apply to the Deep River Science Academy. This is a summer program that engages high school students in research opportunities for credit

✓ Outward Bound runs expeditions (canoeing, kayaking, climbing, snowshoeing) for which high school students can get either a single credit or full semester of credit

Extracurricular

Doctors tend to be well-rounded people. Being a doctor requires skill in a number of areas, and so those who are solely intellectuals rarely succeed in medicine. It's not unusual to meet a doctor who also plays a musical instrument, is a marathon runner, or is highly involved in student government. The opportunities to develop your well-roundedness in high school are endless. You will never again in your life have the amount of free time to expand your horizons as you do in high school. Try new things, find something you like, and don't be afraid to do something uncharacteristic. If you're artistic, by all means participate in the art show, but also try out for a sports team. Try to find a way to be involved both through school and in your community. I would recommend trying a number of different activities, but also try to sustain your involvement over a number of years. Remember that you can participate in extracurricular activities during the summer as well as during the school year. The time commitment could vary anywhere from two hours each week for a few years to a rather frequent yet condensed one-month experience.

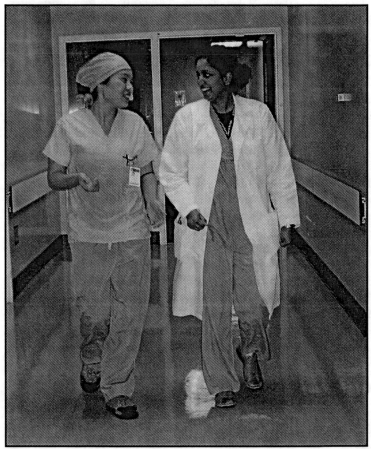

Two first-year residents on their way to rounds

Volunteer

There's a huge range of volunteer activities available while in high school. Again, the important thing is to find something you like, something you feel is actually beneficial to someone else, and something you can learn from. The skills you take on as a volunteer often overlap with other areas of extracurricular development. Being a girl guide leader could, for example, be considered to be leadership involvement, and coaching a soccer team could be seen as both athletics and volunteering. There are many community and school organizations that are looking for volunteers, and there is a niche for you.

Volunteering does not have to be through a pre-organized group, although there are definitely benefits to having a schedule and some goals already provided. Volunteering can be finding a need in your community and filling it. This type of volunteer work may develop your skills even more, as you need to identify the issue, organize a solution, and respond to the needs of your group of interest. This can require a great deal of leadership ability. This may be as simple as regularly giving your time to an elderly neighbour, or as grand as undertaking the development of an after-school daycare program for children of single parents.

I'd recommend keeping a journal in high school, to help you reflect on your experiences. It will help you discover who you are, what you enjoy, and what you want to do with yourself. It's also advisable to start a CV, listing your activities, your hours spent, what you learned from each activity, and the name and contact information of someone who supervised you. You'll find this base CV useful not only when applying to medical school, but also when applying for jobs, scholarships, and special extracurricular opportunities.

Keeping your options open:

Try new things, but don't do anything stupid. You may be required to disclose a criminal record when applying to medical school. Enough said.

Choosing a University

There are many factors to consider when choosing a university and program. Whatever your choice, you need to feel comfortable in the environment. Look for a university that offers the courses that will be prerequisites for medical school. Each university has a different reputation. When you're applying to medical school, though, the university you attended is not taken into account. Because the schools themselves are not weighted, it's important that you go to a university that offers courses that interest you in an environment that inspires you. Take the time to speak to people who are currently attending different universities, and go to the university open houses and speak with a guidance councillor about your academic aspirations. You're going to be spending a number of years at university; and it's worth it to make an informed decision.

Doc Talk

I did a four-year undergrad in physiology, but I didn't start there because I didn't do a science-oriented grade 12. I actually did an IB program, so I wasn't able to apply directly to a science program. But I was able to take some science courses as electives and then apply to the science program.

—Midori Yamamoto, 4th year medical student

There are a few different strategies that people employ when applying to university with medicine in mind:

1) Apply to a school with a good reputation, which will be more difficult to get into:

Pro: You'll probably get a good overall education, excellent libraries, and access to professors doing interesting research. If you're not accepted to medical school it may be easier to continue with a graduate program. If you do not get into medical school, your degree holds a little more authority when applying for other jobs. There are likely to be ample opportunities for extracurricular activities at such schools.

Con: The grading scheme at these prestigious schools can deflate your marks, and you may be able to achieve higher grades elsewhere. The medical school application does not discriminate based on which undergraduate university you attended, and the marks are not adjusted upward if you attended a more difficult university. Marks are a big part of the medical school application. The atmosphere at many of these schools is often quite competitive, since many people will be applying to medical school. You're less likely to receive a scholarship to attend these universities unless your high school marks are extremely high and your resume is extremely impressive.

2) Apply to a professional healthcare program like nursing or physiotherapy:

Pro: You'll graduate with a degree that allows you to work in the field of healthcare. You're guaranteed to spend time working with patients, even if you're not accepted at medical school.

Con: The program may be more structured and it may be more difficult to take courses outside the curriculum, and these courses are required if you wish to apply to medical school. You may need to do these during the summer or only apply to medical schools that do not have these required courses. You may also need to justify your change from one professional program to another on your medical school application.

3) Go to a less demanding, or easier undergraduate university:

Pro: If you have very high marks in high school, then you may be offered a scholarship to attend an easier undergraduate university. This will alleviate some of the financial burden, and can be seen as an achievement in its own right. Your marks may be higher at this university than at a more difficult university.

Con: There may be fewer research opportunities, especially if it's primarily an undergraduate university. Your degree may not carry as much weight when applying for jobs or other opportunities if you do not get into medical school or decide to pursue a different career.

4) Attend a Northern Ontario university (Laurentian or Lakehead) to achieve Northern Status if you don't already have it:

Pro: The Northern Ontario Medical School has location of residence as a major determining factor in choosing its medical class. Attending a Northern Ontario school counts as having a rural or Northern community as your place of residence.

Con: This is probably not enough criteria on which to pick a school where you'll spend the next three or four years.

5) Choose a school where you feel happy, where you can visualise yourself living for the next three or four years, and where the courses that interest you can be taken:

This should override any other strategy. If you're not happy with your school, you'll do miserably and have a rotten university experience. It's hard to be miserable and do well enough in school to be accepted into medical school, or into any program for that matter!

What If I Didn't Know I Wanted to Become a Doctor Back Then?

You do not have to decide to become a doctor while you're still in high school. In fact, I would discourage you from making the "medicine or bust" decision until you're at least in university. High school is a time for exploration. If you're considering medicine and want to make your time in high school beneficial to future applications, then good for you; but don't rule out other careers at this point. In fact, participating in a number of activities and getting good grades in high school not only prepares you for medicine, but also a number of other careers. Your experiences will hopefully expose you to careers you may have not considered otherwise. This will help you make an educated decision about your future.

Many people make the decision to apply to medicine later in life— after university, graduate school, or after training for and working in another field. The experiences you have as an adult in the years prior to medical school are extremely important. Starting to prepare for medicine in high school can help set you on the path to medicine, but it's not the only path. Fear not!

Personal goals during High School

✓ Do well in school
✓ Develop a sense of self
✓ Give of yourself
✓ Get something out of your experiences
✓ Try things that force you to grow
✓ Learn who you are and become aware of your strengths and weaknesses
✓ Spend time with people who are different than you and learn from them
✓ Do something physical
✓ Do something artistic
✓ Try on the leadership role
✓ Keep a diary
✓ Try to imagine yourself in the future
✓ Make some mistakes and learn from them
✓ Go somewhere new
✓ Participate in a co-op program
✓ Take on an interesting summer job
✓ Find a need in your community and fill it
✓ Find interesting ways to complete your high school coursework
✓ Take a course that's nothing like your other courses
✓ Don't drop math
✓ Go above and beyond
✓ Learn to be honest with yourself
✓ Apply for university

For University Students

University is the time period that most people start conscientiously working towards entrance into medical school. It's also the time that many straight-A high school students first realize how stiff the competition is to get into medical school. The way your time is spent during university will greatly influence your ability to get into medical school, in that it's your undergraduate grades that are most often used as the initial cut-off criteria.

Take courses that interest you. There's no single path to medical school; I know people who've come from a variety of backgrounds, including English, engineering, law, and geology, and have still found their way to medicine. However, many medical schools require that you take biology, calculus, chemistry, organic chemistry, physics, and English to apply. You'll also need these courses to write the MCAT. If you're seriously applying, you'll want to cast your net as far as possible, and it would be a shame if you weren't able to apply somewhere just because you didn't take the prerequisite courses. So, if you want to take history in your undergraduate years, do it, especially if you're not yet sure about what you want to do with your life. If you're thinking about medicine, take at least the courses needed to get in. So, plan ahead!

Extracurricular

Universities are filled with clubs for every personality type. Personally, I think it would be a good idea to see if you can continue doing something you enjoyed during high school, but with more responsibility, greater challenge, and a higher level of skill. First of all, it's nice when you're in a new environment to have a sense of continuity in your life, which will make the transition in general easier. As a bonus, it's good to show that you're able to both commit to something and grow with it. In addition, I would suggest trying something completely new and different from your coursework and old activities. It's good for your soul to branch out and put yourself in a position where you have to stretch a little, and it gives you more of a chance to get to know yourself. So, take up kickboxing or rock climbing, or audition for that play!

Social

You need some time to unwind, relax, veg out, and really nurture your social relationships. An absolute minimum is one night a week. I'm sure you'll find time for more. It's very easy to become obsessed with applying to medical school. It can seem like nothing else matters and that if you don't get in the world will stop turning and your life will be over. And the more you work towards medical school, the more invested you become, and the more accountable you feel because friends and family around you know, which can further increase the pressure you put on yourself to get in. It's not a huge leap from being extremely committed to being absolutely nutty. If you find yourself thinking about nothing but preparing for medical school, take a step back and re-assess what you're doing with yourself and how you're spending your time. By making sure you continue to see your friends and family you'll feel more relaxed, be able to put things in perspective, and probably be a more interesting person to be around.

Research

I would highly suggest some sort of research experience if you can get it. It's preferable to work with an M.D. Start asking around a department that interests you before December. This may require writing letters.

Participating in research is a great experience from a career-exploration point of view. By spending some time in the medical field, it can help you decide if you really enjoy biomedical problem solving. Any type of clinical research will give you a better feel for this than bench research, but even bench research can expose you to the types of questions asked in medicine and the environment in which they are asked. It also gives you the opportunity to see if you enjoy research and if you would actually prefer it as a career. Research also provides some definite advantages when it comes to applying to medical school. Researching takes a certain amount of intellectual ability and creativity. It also requires perseverance. Participating in research can act as proof that you either have or are developing these skills. You may get to work with a physician, which would give you an opportunity to find out more about what doctors do. You may get to present your findings in a paper, poster, or at a conference. This is considered a bonus on any medical school application. If you did clinical research, it's a great example of your ability to work with patients. If your supervisor likes your work, they would be in a great position to write you a letter of recommendation.

Your Summers

This is the prime time to get experiences you need to make sure you're choosing the right career, to live and explore a little, and to show that you have what it takes to succeed in medicine.

Volunteer

If you have the luxury of volunteering (that is, if you don't need a paying job) find something that amazes and inspires you. It's easier to be passionate about working with real people in a small organisation than about licking envelopes in a large, well-known organisation. For your own sake and sanity, do volunteer work that's meaningful to *you*, not what you think will be meaningful to an admissions committee. University is a great time of your life when you're old enough to do amazing, independent, and unique things, but often still young enough not to have acquired too many commitments. University summers are four months long, which is plenty of time in which to get something done. Therefore, if you ever wanted to spend a summer categorizing endangered plants in Costa Rica, building houses with Habitat for Humanity, or wanted to start your own food bank, university summers are the time to do it.

Cool Jobs

Yes, they're out there.

See if you can combine a job with international experience, such as teaching English overseas, being an au pair, or being a camp counsellor in another country.

See if you can start your own business. If you're the entrepreneurial type, the Ontario government will provide loans for start-up costs for small businesses run by students. See what types of opportunities there are working in an environment where you're interacting with and helping people such as at a zoo, science centre, nursing home, foster home, or camp.

Your university years are pivotal as to whether or not you'll get into medical school.

Major Tasks to Complete in University

Year One: Get into an academic program you enjoy. Start taking first-year medical school prerequisites. Participate in extracurricular activities that interest you. Find a summer job volunteer work that is satisfying and hopefully helps you decide if you like working in the medical field. Research medical schools that you might want to apply to.

Year Two: Maintain good grades. Take the rest of your prerequisite courses. Study for and take the MCAT. Try not to become obsessive.

Year Three: Decide whether or not to apply to medical school at the beginning of the year. Only your first two years of grades will be considered during this application. Continue to work hard academically, because if you do not get in, your third-year marks will show up on your next application (submitted in year four). Continue in activities that you enjoy and that help you to grow. Consider taking on a leadership role. Make sure you continue to spend time with friends and family. If you need to re-take the MCAT, do it during the summer after your third year. Start thinking about a backup plan. Consider approaching people who might be willing to provide good references for you.

Year Four: Apply to medical school (perhaps again). Keep up your marks. If your backup plan includes applying to graduate school or other programs, make sure you find out what's required for these early on. Stay up-to-date with current events, participate in practice interviews, and buy or borrow a suit. Maintain worthy friendships.

Doc Talk

I had a close friend that I could chat with and be honest with. She helped me to realize what I had done that was valuable. It's sometimes hard to think insightfully about your experiences.
                    –Dr. Rickesh Sood, 2nd year family medicine resident

I worked with seniors in a veterans' hospital. I worked at a chemotherapy treatment centre. I worked with my church taking care of the lawn. All those little things that you think don't count, they add up. I always chose things I enjoyed, but they were always geared towards getting into medical school.

–Dr. Sandra DeMontbrun, 3rd year general surgery resident

For Graduate Students

So, you're a graduate student. You've taken the time to go beyond a basic undergraduate education and are now considering medical school. Maybe you started out thinking you wanted to do academic work, but now think you want to change direction. Maybe this was your plan all along and you wanted to try research before deciding if medicine was really for you. Maybe you've already applied to medical school and are working towards a graduate degree as your backup plan. Perhaps you didn't know what you wanted to do with your life when you graduated from university and this seemed like a good way to stay on top of things without venturing into the workforce. Regardless of your reasons for starting graduate school, if you're enrolled in a graduate program, either a masters or a PhD, there are many pros and a few cons when applying to medical school.

On the pro side, you're probably more mature than applicants coming out of undergraduate school. You've had more years to do more stuff. You've been able to work more, travel more, had more opportunities to join clubs, volunteer, experience more, and reflect on things. You probably have a better idea of who you are and what you want out of life. Moreover, maybe you have already applied to medical school, which gives you an advantage when it comes to organizing your applications and preparing for your interview.

Graduate school itself can also be an advantage. You'll have had the opportunity to do research, present at conferences, and perhaps even publish something or teach a class. All of these things will definitely add to the personal characteristics, extracurricular activities, and academic achievement portions of your application.

If your research enabled you to interact with patients, you will have had experience both working with patients and doing research.

However, all those A's you get in graduate school do not always increase your academic average. For the most part, your undergraduate grades will haunt you, even if you're doing a PhD and it's been six years since you took an undergraduate course. Each school has its own policy when it comes to how to treat graduate students applying to medical school. Some schools will consider some of your graduate school marks at a certain weight if your undergraduate marks meet a certain cut-off point. Some schools will add points to your application score. Others have a separate committee that evaluates graduate students on grades and publication productivity. Please see the appendix for the specifics of each school.

Another caveat for graduate students: many schools will not accept applications from graduate students who've not yet finished their degree. If you start a two year masters program, you might not be able to apply to medical school until you're in your final year, meaning you'll have to take a year off between application cycles. Likewise, if you're halfway through a PhD, some schools will not accept your application until you're done, and you may need to wait four or five years before applying again! Not all schools have this policy, but it does decrease the pool of schools to which you can apply. Most schools also require that your supervisor send them a letter. This letter should confirm your supervisor's awareness of your application to the school in question, and should also reveal when your supervisor believes your research will be complete. This makes it hard to say to your supervisor, "Yes! I'd love to start my PhD in your lab," and be applying to medical school on the side.

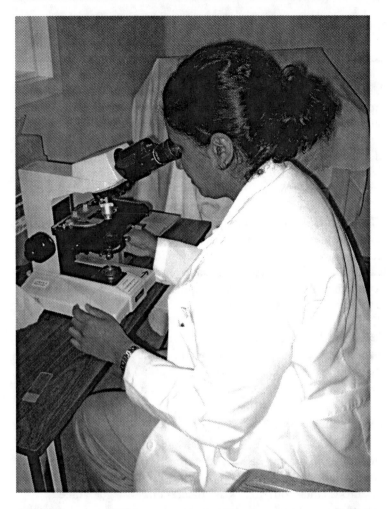

Applying to medical school after a graduate degree gives you
time to explore your options and build on your experiences.

For Aboriginal Students

Aboriginal students are extremely underrepresented in medicine.
There are a number of complicated factors that contribute to this
disparity, and many medical schools are working to make medical
education more accessible to Aboriginal students. Some schools, such
as Saskatchewan, have a medical mentorship program to expose

interested Aboriginal youth to medicine as a career. The new Northern Ontario School of Medicine has admission criteria that take into account living in the north or having a strong connection to the north, so if you live or have lived in a northern community, then you may have an advantage at this school. The curriculum of this school was created in collaboration with the Aboriginal communities in the area, and encourages Aboriginal students to consider medicine.

Many schools reserve seats for Aboriginal applicants. If you're applying as an Aboriginal applicant (it is not necessary to identify yourself as an Aboriginal applicant unless you want to), the GPA or MCAT requirements may be different than the standard application pool. The admissions process may be more heavily weighted towards your participation in the community or the interview. Other schools require the same GPA cut-off, but offer an interview to all Aboriginal applicants. Most schools will require a letter of support from your band council, treaty, community, or organization. Some schools also ask for additional essays and other information.

Please see the appendix at the back for specifics regarding admissions requirements. I encourage you to call the schools to enquire about extra packages or forms.

Finances

Medical school is expensive, but money should not be a factor in your decision to apply. Although it's expensive, if you plan well you'll not run into financial difficulties. Medical school is a guaranteed investment in your brain. You have to put the money in, and it will be a long time before you see any financial return (approximately ten years). You will make enough in the end to pay off your loans. You just have to be ready to take that leap.

Tuition alone costs approximately $15,000 per year, which is not the kind of money that most people have available to them. There are also the very real costs of books, equipment, travel expenses, rent, an Internet connection, and a professional wardrobe. It will be next to impossible to have a job during medical school, and although some people are able to work during the first two summers, many choose to use the time to do research or extra clinical work. Do not fear, though - although these expenses are large, they're not insurmountable, and money is available to you.

Expenses in Medical School

This is a general list of expenses you'll need to cover while you're in medical school. The list will vary from person to person, depending on variables such as the city in which you live and personal spending habits.

ONE TIME EXPENDITURES

Equipment (e.g., stethoscope)	$ 500
Computer	$ 1,000
Palm Pilot	$ 400
TOTAL	$ 1,900

YEARLY EXPENSES

Tuition	$15,000
Transportation	$ 1,500
Business Wardrobe	$ 300
Books	$ 500
TOTAL YEARLY EXPENSES	$17,300

MONTHLY EXPENSES

Rent	$ 800
Utilities	$ 100
Food	$ 250
Parking	$ 100
TOTAL MONTHLY EXPENSES	$ 1,250

OTHER MISCELLANEOUS EXPENSES
Travel expenses/living expenses during electives: $3,000
CaRMS application fees and interviewing expenses: $6,000
LMCC Part I: $1,000

Sources of Money

1) Canadian student loans and provincial student loans

These are usually quite generous. If you've been living away from your parents for at least four years (as most people have by the time they begin medical school) their parent's income will not be taken into account when calculating the amount of loan available to you.

Due to the size of the loan, you may also be eligible for the Canada millennium bursary. If you need a car for medical school, see if you can keep it in your parents' name instead of your own, since part of the car's value will be held against the amount of loan for which you'll be eligible. You'll need to start paying off your debt when you being your residency unless you do your residency at Memorial in Newfoundland.

2) Bursaries from your medical school

To receive a bursary, most often you must have applied to Canada Student Loans and provincial student loans. So even if you don't think you'll receive anything from these loans, it's worth applying for so you're eligible for bursaries. Keep in mind that you will have to claim bursaries as income when you do your taxes.

3) Banks

Banks want to give large loans to get students through medical school. Unless you have a rich uncle who has been stashing money between his mattresses so you could go to medical school, you'll likely need to apply for a line of credit with a bank. Because you're in medical school, you'll often only be charged the prime rate (as opposed to the prime rate plus 1% or 2%) as interest. These lines of credit are around $150,000, and you're charged interest only on the amount that you take out. Most people I know had to take out a line of credit to make it through medical school. The Canadian and provincial loans only really cover tuition, if that.

4) The Canadian Armed Forces

If you're willing to become a family physician and are not limited to a single geographic area, you might consider joining the armed forces while in medical school. The armed forces cover books, tuition, and equipment. In addition, the Canadian Forces pay a yearly salary to students while in medical school. They also offer a fairly significant signing bonus. While in medical school, you have the rank of second lieutenant, and as a resident, you have the rank of lieutenant. In return, you must choose family medicine as your residency, and you're required to provide four years of service to the armed forces. You'll likely be working at a base in Canada for the majority of the time. However, you can be deployed anywhere the armed forces are deployed, and therefore it's likely that you'll spend approximately six months of your return-of-duty time overseas. There are opportunities for extra training in the areas of general and orthopaedic surgery, anaesthesiology, internal medicine, radiology, and psychiatry. However, there is mandatory service agreement of years on top of the initial four.

I used the following websites to research this section. I recommend that you read them yourself or contact the Canadian Forces if you think this option might work for you.

http://64.254.158.112/pdf/MOTP_en.pdf
http://www.forces.ca/v3/engraph/jobs/jobs.aspx?id=55&bhcp=1

The Bottom Line

Money really is there to get you through medical school. There's no reason why only those with money already in the bank should be applying. Do not let money issues stop you from pursuing this dream. Things will be tighter for you if you have a partner or children, but hopefully will not be impossible. If you already have student debt, you'll be able to put the payments for it on hold while you're enrolled full-time in a university program.

The caveat: Even though you have a large line of credit available, you must still be cautious with your spending. Interest adds up quickly. When you graduate from medical school your starting salary will be the equivalent of minimum wage for the first year, when calculated by the hour. You may want to reserve part of that line of credit for a down payment on a house or to help you with expenses during your first year of residency. Remember you'll be making payments on your student loans during this year as well.

If you think you need one, get a financial advisor. The Canadian Medical Association has financial advisors available to all medical students as part of their membership. These financial advisors do not represent any particular bank or loaning institution, and their sole purpose is to help doctors manage their money. They'll be able to give you unbiased advice regarding finances.

PART III: MEDICAL SCHOOL

"I would sit on my porch every day waiting for the letter. The postman knew that I was waiting for the letter. I would get on my bike and go up and down the street waiting to see if he was coming. I remember getting that 8-by-10-inch brown envelope. It was thin. I remember opening it up and reading it really quickly. When it said I was accepted, I started to cry. I was jumping up and down. It was one of the best days of my life. I still have that acceptance letter and there's a blotch of smudged ink from a teardrop. It's so clear in my mind. I remember running down the hall, sitting at the table to read it again, slipping with my socks on the hardwood floor. I remember every little second. It was the best feeling. It was like getting engaged or finding out you're going to have a baby. All those years of work, of studying, preparing for the MCAT, the social things you had to give up – it's all lifted because you got in. It's the best thing ever. We ordered in Chinese food and invited all the neighbors."
—Dr. Sandra DeMontbrun, 3rd Year General Surgery Resident

CHAPTER 9: THE PRECLINICAL YEARS

CONGRATULATIONS, you've made it! You've beaten the odds and earned a seat in a Canadian Medical School. The next three or four years will be some of the most wonderful, stressful, and eye-opening years of your life. The time goes by quickly, so enjoy medicine in this protected environment while you can. Read often, ask questions, and see every single patient you can. Residency is closer than you think!

Doc Talk

Medical school was a culture shock for me because I went from the workforce and a masters, both of which were very flexible, to an undergraduate program (medicine), which had no flexibility at all.
–Dr. Jennifer Graham, 1ˢᵗ year paediatric resident

Would You Just Have a Look at this Rash for Me?

When you receive that juicy package in the mail, you'll notice something peculiar start to happen. People will want your medical advice. Even before you know anything about anything, you'll be asked a number of personal medical questions.

First of all, don't let it go to your head.

Second, there's nothing wrong with sharing information, but I wouldn't actually give medical advice. If fact, even after you become a doctor you should refrain from providing medical advice in a casual manner. Even offering this casual advice enters you into a doctor-patient relationship, and with it comes many responsibilities. You cannot properly examine a patient at a cocktail party, or ask all the questions you might want to. The person might not feel they can respond truthfully because they don't want others to overhear, or do not want to share a certain piece of personal information with you. If a friend were to ask me for medical advice about her knee pain outside a healthcare setting, I may say, "I can't give you advice because I can't properly assess you. However, if you're asking about the problem in general, here's some information. This doesn't necessarily refer to you, and if you're worried you should see your family doctor."

It's always appropriate, responsible, and ethical to respond to an emergency situation to the best of your ability. Responding to an emergency situation always involves calling 911 and getting help.

Problem-Based Learning

Problem-Based Learning (PBL) is an educational concept where, instead of just listening to lectures about medicine, you participate in discussion groups and learn medicine "around" a paper patient. You'll be presented with a clinical scenario, and it's your job to discover what questions need to be asked and then find the answers to those questions. The small group PBL sessions are supplemented by lectures and clinical skills teaching.

PBL is a technique used in a many medical schools worldwide, including Harvard (USA), University of Sydney (Australia), and Manchester (England).

The following Canadian Medical Schools use a PBL or modified PBL curriculum:

Dalhousie
Ottawa
McMaster

Toronto
Queens
Western
Northern Ontario
University of Alberta

Many people find that this promotes self-study skills and a deeper understanding of the issues. The relevance of the material you're learning is also more apparent.

Each case results in the development of a list of learning objectives, which are completed and discussed at the next meeting. For example, you might get the case: "Mr. H is a sixty-four-year-old man who works as a mechanic. Over the past few years, he's noticed that he sometimes feels some aching in his chest when he's working. He's never been to a doctor about it and he assumes it's nothing more than heartburn. One day, while lifting a box of equipment at the garage, the pain intensifies and he feels nauseated. He drops the box and falls to the ground. A co-worker sees what's happened and calls 911. The ambulance arrives ten minutes later, and the attendants see Mr. H still lying on the ground. He's sweating and complaining of intense pressure in his chest. The attendants find his vitals to be as follows:

O2 sats 95%
BP 110/68
HR 90
RR 24
Temp 37°

This case may go on to discuss what happens at the hospital, lab values, clinical findings, treatment options, etc.

After reading the case, you and your group brainstorm issues. These may be:

What are the signs and symptoms of a heart attack?
What else could present as a heart attack?
Who is most likely to have a heart attack?
What types of heart attacks are there?
What is the anatomy of the heart?

How do the medications that are used to treat or prevent heart attacks work?

What community resources are available for people with heart disease?

How do share bad news to family members?

What are the initial emergency steps you take if you suspect someone is having a heart attack?

What is tryponin?

What is angina?

What are normal cholesterol values?

After brainstorming with your group, you condense the issues into a few clear objectives. For example:

1. review the anatomy of the heart and the coronary arteries

2. understand the pathophysiology and sequelae of coronary artery disease

3. Discuss treatment options acute MI and when they are used

After the objectives are set, you go off to research these topics using whatever resources are available to you, such as textbooks, online resources, or clinical experts.

When you meet again, you discuss the topics and help each other clarify what you've learned.

I suggest you read the following articles about PBL to learn more about it:

http://bmj.bmjjournals.com/cgi/reprint/326/7384/328.pdf
http://www.mja.com.au/public/issues/may4/schmidt/schmidt.html
http://www.fhs.mcmaster.ca/images/publications/Saturday_Night.pdf
http://meds.queensu.ca/medicine/pbl/pblhome.htm

The Social Aspect and Extracurricular Activities

Believe it or not, even though you're in medical school there's still time to get out and participate in extracurricular activities. In fact, the vast majority of people do. Medical school is sometimes like an intimate slice of university. Many people join clubs that are specifically for medical students, ranging from rock climbing clubs, to choirs and water polo teams. There's also the opportunity to get involved in student government at your school level or on a national level. While in medical school, you'll get to know some of the most dynamic and motivated people you'll ever meet. Although the workload is heavy, it's worth enjoying the social and extracurricular activities to keep you from becoming obsessive and one-dimensional. When you're applying to CaRMS you'll be asked about social, leadership, extracurricular, and research activities you participated in during medical school, and this is another good reason why you should undertake as many diverse activities as possible.

Doc Talk

I took classes at art school during medical school. It was just something fun to do. They had an artist-in-residence program. She would hold workshops in the anatomy lab so we could practice drawing in the anatomy lab. We also had a narrative expert, and she held workshops in first year about learning how to tell stories in a way that's interesting. It's a great skill to have.

—Midori Yamamoto, 4th year medical student

Remember, you're not "destined" to be in medicine. There's not just one area of life that you'll succeed in. Don't worry, life's not linear, it's curvilinear. We're almost taught that life is supposed to be linear once you get into medicine. You get in and then you take the right electives to get into the right residency program, and then you want a specific fellowship so you work hard and get that specific fellowship, and then you find a job exactly where you want to work and then you die. It's like a train. When are you going to get off that train and say, "enough?" You can take time off during medical school and explore other things.

—Dr. Rickesh Sood, 2nd year family medicine resident

In medical school, I learned how to play hockey and ultimate Frisbee and I sang in the choir and the beer bottle orchestra. I tried a whole bunch of things I had never tried before. You have to have friends on the inside of medicine to survive.

—Dr. Jennifer Graham, 1st year paediatrics resident

Should I Work During Medical School?

The workload and challenges of medical school are generally prohibitive when it comes to having a job. This doesn't mean that it's impossible, and I know that some people are able to work a part-time job at certain points during medical school. If you have dependents, you'll probably be especially interested in this option. I did not work during medical school. The people I knew who did work tended to have jobs for which they were already qualified, which allowed them to work unconventional hours (not nine in the morning to five at night), and were flexible. Some former nurses worked a few shifts as such, and I knew a pharmacist who would work a few weekends during the day at a local drugstore. I also knew a student who was already involved in teaching some tutorials at the university who managed to continue this line of work during medical school. Although this is possible in the pre-clinical years, it becomes fairly impractical when you start your clinical clerkship, when your time will no longer be your own. You will be subject to a call schedule over which you will almost certainly have no control. You will be on call one of every four days, and your weekly schedule will be varied and unpredictable. During this time in your training things like sleeping, studying, and leisure time are at a premium. In general, I would recommend against working, unless you're really in need of work from a financial perspective. Your plate will be quite full already, and you will need to be able to focus on learning without worrying if you will be able to find someone to cover your shift.

If you're attending a four-year medical school, you may have an opportunity to work during the summers between those first three years. Many people choose to use this time to prepare for residency by doing research, volunteer activities, or clinical work associated with their area of interest. If you do need some income, you might still be able to expand your medical horizons at the same time. There are many funded research spots if you're willing to look for them. Some rural electives will also provide funding for the duration of your time. In the end, you have to decide how your time is best spent. How badly do you need the money? Can you find a funded position that matches your interests? Is there a special opportunity that you can't pass up? Is it worth your while to participate even if you will not make any money?

Do You Need a Car?

You may need to consider the major expenditure of purchasing a car before you begin medical school. Call the school or ask students in the program if they've needed one. Some hospitals are quite spread out in certain cities, and the only way to efficiently travel between them may be to drive. Many programs also make use of community hospitals that could be some distance from where you'll be living, requiring you to commute daily or even live in another city during this time period.

Depending on your program, you may only need a car during clerkship. This will mean you can delay the purchase until then, which will also delay the associated auto expenses such as parking, insurance, and car payments. When possible, register the car in your parents' name, since the value of your car will be considered an asset when you apply for student loans. Read the student loan policy carefully to see how much you'll be penalized for owning a car.

There are alternatives to owning an automobile. Perhaps you only need a car occasionally or during a specific rotation. If your need is infrequent enough, it might be cheaper to take a taxi, a rental car, or another form of public transportation on the rare occasion that you need to go somewhere, rather than paying for a car and all its monthly expenses when you may only use it three times in a year.

Talk to people and find out what your real transportation needs are. Keep in mind that as a medical student, your mode of transportation needs to be flexible and reliable. The hours you'll be working and attending classes are untraditional hours. Would you feel comfortable waiting at a bus stop at eleven thirty at night to go home? If you're on call from home, will you be able to get to the hospital in a timely fashion if you're called in to see a patient or assist in a surgery?

Are there fewer buses and subway trains on weekends or after five at night? Do buses start running in time for you to be in the hospital to round at six in the morning?

Remember to make arrangements to get yourself home post call other than driving yourself. Residents have a greater chance of being in a car accident while driving at this time. Stay and sleep, arrange for someone to pick you up, or just take a taxi.

CHAPTER 10: TESTING

MEDICAL students write tests that are similar to those you have written in undergraduate classes. Some are multiple-choice, and some require written answers (long answer). However, there are two types of tests that new medical students are probably unfamiliar with—the oral exam and the Objective Structured Clinical Examination (OSCE).

The Oral Exam

Oral examinations usually involve a thirty to sixty minute interaction between you and one or more staff person. Sometimes you'll be asked to present a case and then are asked questions surrounding the case. Other times you'll be presented with a clinical situation and then are asked questions around it. The oral exam tests your clinical skills with questions like, "A patient shows up in the emergency room complaining of right upper quadrant pain, vomiting, and fever. What else would you want to know on history and physical exam, and what labs would you order?" You may also be asked a more theory-based question such as, "What stimulates the gall bladder to contract?" Other theory-based questions might include, "How does Warfarin work?" or "What are the risk factors for coronary artery disease?"

During an oral exam, any topic that you mention yourself (either during the case study or as part of your answer) is generally fair game for additional questions. The questioning continues along a certain line of thinking until you are no longer able to answer them. When you feel you have reached this point in the questioning, it is much better to say that you don't know than to fabricate an answer.

I prepared for oral examinations by making sure I had my case-study well rehearsed, and read material around all of the aspects of the case. For example, if a patient in your case has a gastric ulcer, make sure you know the classic presentation, appropriate work-up including the "gold standard" for diagnosis, etiology, treatments, side-effects of treatment, and success rates. If during your case your patient needs fluid resuscitation, make sure you know how to calculate appropriate amounts of fluid, what types of fluids are available, and what you should be monitoring during fluid resuscitation.

These types of exams can be extremely intimidating. It would be wise to try to find some examples of oral exam scenarios to practice with.

The Objective Structured Clinical Examination (OSCE)

The OSCE is the classic medical school examination. It's used to test your actual "doctoring skills" by providing a standardized patient (an actor who pretends to have a certain ailment) and your clinical skills are judged by a physician-examiner who watches you perform. There are multiple stations with a standardized patient behind each door. You're usually given between one and two minutes to read a statement about the situation, after which you are given ten minutes to "do what doctors do" during the patient examination. Sometimes the situation is social instead of clinical, such as a woman making an appointment with you because she found out you prescribed her teenaged daughter birth control pills. Sometimes the patient will be angry, depressed, manic, or suffering from dementia. Some patients are there just for clinical examination, where you are simply instructed to conduct an appropriate examination of the knee. There really is something different behind each door. At times, you'll be given an X-ray or an EKG to interpret instead of having a patient. You'll always get points for introducing yourself appropriately, and washing your hands before you start. The whole exam often takes over two hours to do, and really is exhausting. I prepared by doing practice tests of this type with my friends. Three people are the perfect number to study with. One person should be the examiner, one can be the patient, and the other can take the test. Then rotate jobs. Find any copies of old OSCEs; they'll be extremely valuable.

How Important are Marks?

Doc Talk

I felt there was actually less stress in medical school than in undergraduate school. I did my undergrad in very medicine-based subjects, so it gave me confidence when I was approaching my medical subjects.

–Midori Yamamoto, 4th year Medical Student

The grading system in the majority of medical schools is quite different from that of university. You're no longer pushing to get the 92% instead of the 88%. Most schools are either pass or fail; or honours, pass, or fail. Some schools may also write specific comments about you on your transcript. Your evaluation in the pre-clerkship period may consist of exams, small group-work, clinical skills, and projects. Your marks during clerkship are also often in the pass or fail format. My medical school transcript reads similarly to my senior kindergarten transcript: "Anne was enthusiastic about her general surgery rotation. She asks appropriate questions and gets along well with other members of the healthcare team." The good part about this type of grading is that your transcript is more likely to reflect any special strengths that you have. Stating that you had an excellent relationship with patients is much more meaningful and specific than the number seventy-eight. Do you work hard? Are you good at it? Are you easy to get along with? Generally, it's your overall performance, and not one specific exam that matters. You can't tuck yourself away and then do well on the final exam to succeed. You need to make a good all-round impression that will read well on your transcript and set you up to ask for letters of recommendation for residency.

CHAPTER 11: THE CLINICAL YEARS—CLERKSHIP!

"The important thing is to make the lesson of each case tell on your education."
—*Sir William Osler*

Little Fish in a Big Pond

THE night before my first day of clerkship I was so excited and nervous that I couldn't sleep. I really felt like things were finally starting. I'll be honest—initially it was overwhelming. You have a name tag and a stethoscope around your neck, so on the outside, you look just like a doctor, and to any patient you may have just as easily been practising for ten years as you have for ten minutes. You have patients that you round on everyday. You try to keep up with what's going on. People are using shorthand that you don't understand, and the handwriting in the charts is frankly impossible to read. Nurses are asking you for orders of drugs you aren't familiar with, and then you feel useless because you need them co-signed anyway. You take hundreds if not thousands of histories and physicals. Sometimes you get a sense of disappointment from your patients when they realize that you're a medical student and they still need to wait for the "real" doctor to get there.

Residents will send you on bizarre hunts through the hospital to find out the results of an MRI on a patient that you haven't even met. You'll be worried that things are happening without you, and you'll therefore follow your resident around so closely that before you know it, you've found yourself mistakenly in the boy's bathroom (and that's not a good thing if you're not a boy). After coming to the startling realisation that for your dignity's sake (and the boy's) you must back off, you decide not to follow your resident quite so closely, only to later discover that you missed scrubbing in on an interesting surgery.

During this time, you'll meet some of the most amazing people in the world. You'll have the time available to actually sit and listen to people's life stories, something that you won't always have as much time for as a resident. You'll walk home late at night stunned from the tragedies and triumphs of the day. Friends outside the world of medicine will assume you spend your days saving lives, but you'll be questioning whether you made each patient's day a little bit better or a little bit worse. When I was a clerk, I often joked, "I'm not a real doctor, I just play one in the hospital." Just remember, Little Fish, this pond is an ocean, and you're only at the very beginning of things. There are years and years ahead of you to try to make sense of it all. A big goal that you should have for the end of your clerkship is to be able to tell whether or not someone is sick. It seams simple, but this is an essential skill that does take time to develop. At the end of your clerkship, you should be able to tell if you need to call for help right away, if it looks like things are slowly heading in an unfavourable direction, or if someone appears to be on the mend. You'll be able to make this assessment after doing thousands of histories and physicals and seeing what people at various stages of those who are sick and those who are not sick look like. So, learn to be safe by learning to know when to call for help. And don't let those who are overworked, tired, and overly confident make you feel like you aren't measuring up to being a big fish. You'll be there one day.

What is a Clerk?

A clerk is a medical student who's doing the clinical aspect of medical school. It's a confusing name, and if you use it to introduce yourself, you will often be mistaken for someone with an administrative role. Once, early in my clerkship, I introduced myself to a patient as a clerk. He became quite upset when I started asking him questions about his medical history. He thought I was some sort of hospital paper-filer. The title *clinical clerk* is better than just *clerk* but I think the term *medical student* communicates your role more clearly.

As a clerk, you'll be spending most of your time in the hospital as part of a healthcare team. Each rotation is organized differently, but generally, you'll be working with a group of medical practitioners and students to see and treat patients.

Doc Talk

You struggle with the insecurity of not knowing.
It's a fine line between doing too much and doing too little. You get in trouble at both ends.

—Chris McCrossin, 4th year medical student

The best part of medical school is realising the scope of medicine. And even as clerks you're only seeing a fraction of it. And medicine is just so much broader than that. Every rotation is just so different. I'm just wowed by the variety!

—Midori Yamamoto, 4th year medical student

Seeing the clerks come through now that I'm an intern, I see that the anxiety I had is totally normal, and that everyone has it. I don't think clerkship is hard, but your confidence and level of knowledge are just not that great.

—Dr. Rickesh Sood, 2nd year family medicine resident

Clerkship was great and incredibly hard! The first bit was terrifying because the process is so hard. Where are the charts? What does the inside of the chart look like? How do I write a note? What should be in it? And on top of all that, of course, is the medicine.

-Dr. Jennifer Graham, 1st year paediatrics resident

You're Part Of a Team

A combination of some or all of the following people may be on your team:

Clinical clerks or medical students

First-year residents, often referred to as interns or PGY1's (Post Graduate Year1's), or R1's (resident 1's)

Second- or third-year residents, also called junior residents

A fourth- or fifth-year resident, also known as a senior resident or chief.

A fellow (a physician who has finished residency and is doing a fellowship program to train in a sub-specialized field, often acting as junior attending physician)

A staff physician, or attending physician (a physician who has completed residency, has been hired by the hospital, and is ultimately responsible for all the patients on the team)

Tips on Surviving Clerkship

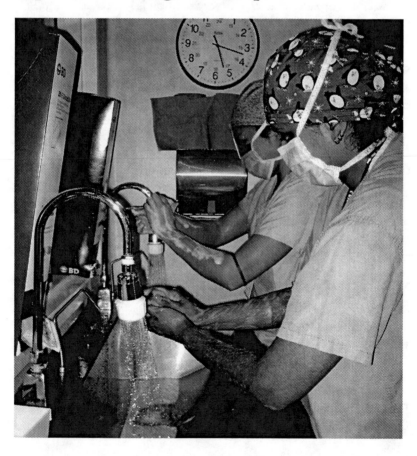

The SuperClerk

Everyone would like to be one. A *SuperClerk* is a mythical creature that requires no sleep, does not need to urinate, can survive without food or water, and can be two places at once. *SuperClerk* always has the correct answer and can see a patient, complete a thorough history, physical, and fill out all preliminary paperwork, all in under seven minutes. *SuperClerk* never minds staying late, memorizes the lab results of all their patients, has never contaminated a sterile field, and cheerfully takes on the same workload as a senior resident. During clerkship you'll at times feel like the expectations are very high—and they are. You're now a member of a healthcare team, and your role is not always clear.

Generally, surviving clerkship is a combination of perseverance and a good attitude. For many people, this will be one of the busiest and most challenging years of their lives (until they become a resident!). There are a few rules that will generally keep you going and maybe nudge you in the direction of the *SuperClerk*:

a. Show up on time. This simple act will show that you're responsible and have respect for your team.

b. At the beginning of a rotation, check in with the team or resident to find out what your schedule is, who you can call, and what your responsibilities are. Some clerks manage to disappear during rotation. These are bad clerks—definitely not SuperClerk-ish.

c. Follow through on what you say you'll do. Keep notes as you walk around. I always put check boxes next to tasks I need to complete.

d. If you don't know, ask. You're new, and it's okay if you don't know how it works. This is your time to figure out what's going on. You'll be much happier asking now as a medical student, rather than when you're alone at eleven at night as a PGY1.

e. Answer your pages promptly. If you don't know how to use the paging system, find out as soon as possible.

f.   See as many patients as you can. You'll be thankful for this the first time you're on call alone as a first-year resident.

g.   Read around your cases. Maybe this should be the first thing on the list! It's too much information to try to follow everything that's happening to the patients on the ward and read a textbook end to end during a rotation. If you see something during the day, or know you'll see the next day, read *that* chapter. You'll then be able to associate a real patient with a story to the information in the textbook, and you'll actually remember it. If, at the end of your rotation, there are still a few things that are important and you didn't see, read about those.

h.   Be helpful. As a medical student, you're just learning your clinical skills, but there are some things that you can do that will earn the respect of residents, staff, and nurses. Clean up after yourself, throw your gloves in the garbage, always dispose of any sharps that you've used after counting them, ask where to put swabs or samples, help with the transport and positioning of patients, help with lifting, and ask what you can do to assist any chance you get.

i.   Try to stay healthy. In the stress of clerkship, many people gain or lose weight depending on their environment. I lost weight during paediatrics (stress of my first rotation, plus gastro I picked up on the ward) and gained it during general surgery (free hot chocolate in the surgeons lounge!).

j.   When it's time to go home, go home. Taking your time off post-call and making use of your vacations will keep you excited and interested in your work.

k.   Carry many pens. You'll make use of a good black pen everyday. As a doctor, your pen is your sword. People will permanently borrow them, leaving you defenseless when the attending asks you to write up orders. Buy a big box of cheap black ballpoint pens and put them in your bag, lab coat, jacket, and anywhere else that will hold a pen.

l.   Yes, when they say you'll be on call one in four they really mean you'll be on call one day out of every four. I'll say it again because I could barely believe it the first time I thought about it. The call is really one in four. This means that every fourth night you'll stay in the hospital until the next day. You do not get to go home in the morning, and you're generally expected to stay until noon. If you start at six in the morning (such as during general surgery) you'll essentially be working a thirty-hour shift. Believe it or not, this is an improvement from what clerkship and residency was like twenty years ago, before there was a Resident's Association. When you get home, you'll be torn between the two necessities of sleeping and eating, wishing you could do both at the same time (caution: my husband insists this is a choking hazard and strongly recommends you choose one over the other). I usually opt for eating and then hit the wall while chewing on a hamburger (post-call indulgence). Finding a way to maintain some semblance of an internal clock is difficult, but possible. I usually nap after my burger anywhere from two to five hours, depending on how rough the night was. Don't over-nap or you'll find it impossible to go to bed on time, setting you up for an exhausting day.

m. When you have the opportunity to do something, do it. When your resident asks if you want to see a patient in the ER, it's a rhetorical question. I had a classmate as a medical student who received a phone call at three in the morning from the resident, who said, "There's a man in the emergency room with chest pain, do you want to go see him?" The student had the gall to say, "No thanks, I already saw a chest pain today." As a medical student, you'll never see enough of a certain type of patient, procedure, or condition to say that you'll gain nothing from seeing or doing something again. Never.

n. Pay attention when someone is doing a presentation. This may sound straight forward, but there are always a few people who take this opportunity to have a private conversation or some who may use the messenger on their PDA during rounds. I know it's very hard, and you may be forgiven if you're post-call, but the person presenting is often a PGY1 or other resident who has put a significant amount of time into the presentation. At least make an attempt at looking interested to avoid being rude.

o. Don't fake being sick. You're surrounded by doctors. Trust me. We know when you're faking it. Faking an illness just makes you look bad and creates more work for everyone else. On the other hand, if you're truly sick, just go home, get better, and don't spread your mucous around.

Doc Talk

When you get a new patient, do their whole history and physical again. It's the only way you'll remember what's going on with them. Sometimes it might feel like a make-work project, or you might feel kind of silly, but then you actually know the patient really well. It's hard when you're coming on and the patient has been there for a while. It's hard to get the story from the chart, especially if they're having a number of investigations going on at the same time. Go through the history, go through the physical, and then go through all the investigations that have been ordered to date. It gives you a picture of what's going on with that patent.

–Chris McCrossin, 4ᵗʰ year medical student

I've really liked my on-call experiences, regardless of what discipline I was in. I've really enjoyed interacting with residents because they're closer to where I am than the staff is. You can pick their minds, their experiences, and ask any questions. I think that's an important part of the clerkship experience.

–Midori Yamamoto, 4ᵗʰ year medical student

The first time I was on call I was doing internal medicine and I was so tired. It was two or three in the morning and the senior wanted to teach. After I presented to him I put my feet up and fell asleep in a chair for maybe twenty minutes. When I woke up, one of the nurses had put a sign on me that said "Do Not Resuscitate." I'll never forget that. Later I was wondering, why is this guy trying to teach me at two or three in the morning? I was holding my head up, trying to keep my eyes open. I remember thinking, oh my God, I'm going to have to do this all night long.

–Dr. Rickesh Sood, 2ⁿᵈ year family medicine resident

I'm used to being good at my job. I earned good money, I did well, and I had contributable skills. Then I went to knowing nothing and really being at the bottom of the ladder. In medicine, you push yourself hard, and you still don't know. Sure, there are times that I'm crying in the stairwells because I am so tired. But that happens maybe once or twice a year, and there are so many amazing times that make up for that.

–Dr. Jennifer Graham, 1ˢᵗ year paediatrics resident

Paediatrics

a. Take care to do everything you can to preserve the family unit. Children are in a strange environment and parents are trusting strangers to care for their children. Do whatever you can to keep the family together.

b. Get to know the families. In paediatrics, you need to respond to the needs and observations of the family. Parents know their children well.

c. If you're overwhelmed, always speak to your Sr.

d. Having a funny sticker on your ID badge or a toy on your stethoscope can really go a long way in terms of distracting a small child when you're trying to examine them.

e. If you suspect abuse, listen to your gut. Speak to your Sr. about how to proceed.

f. Paediatrics is multidisciplinary and everyone is a child advocate. Interact with the social workers, dieticians, nurses, and physiotherapists to better understand your patients' needs.

g. Learn how to hold a baby gently and confidently. It can be very intimidating to examine a very young baby. You'll have a better experience if you're comfortable doing the physical exam.

h. Wash your hands and stethoscope. Kids put their fingers in their nose, touch their sores, and then everything around them. Washing your hands between every patient encounter will protect your patients as well as yourself from infection (I became extremely sick during my paediatric rotation, so did most people I know).

i. Warm up your stethoscope, and if your patient is sleeping or quiet, take the opportunity to listen to everything before they become anxious and start crying.

j. All doses in paediatrics are calculated based on weight. Carry a calculator or a palm pilot with you.

k. Remember that most parents care about their children more than themselves.

Obstetrics and Gynaecology

a. When on labour and delivery call, don't leave the floor. If you're interested in getting hands-on experience delivering babies, you need to be available at all times. When things get going you are not likely to be paged.

b. Trust birth and remember that delivering a baby is something that healthy people do. It's a family event and a joyous occasion. Do whatever you can to maintain an atmosphere of health and make sure your patients feel in control of the birth.

c. If you want to deliver someone's baby, you need to be involved in their care. Don't arrive at the last moment expecting to deliver the head when the mother has been in labour for twelve hours. You should do the admission and check on your patient a minimum of once every two hours.

d. Never do a cervical check unsupervised.

e. Remember that pain is a personal experience. How that pain is managed is the patient's choice and no one else's.

f. Remember that the experience of pain is increased in an anxious environment. You have a duty to the patient to stay calm.

g. Tell the resident that you're keen to meet patients and participate in a hands-on way. Stick around.

h. To do well in gynaecology, get organized before you start any exam, and always be supervised. The only way to learn what you're doing is to practice.

i. In a Gyn OR, as in any OR, you should meet the patient before you're involved in their surgery.

j.   Become comfortable asking questions about partner abuse. If your gut tells you that something's wrong or if something is revealed to you, talk to your Sr. about it.

k.   Wear comfortable, closed, waterproof shoes. Obstetrics and gynaecology can get very wet. I've personally had to throw away a good pair of running shoes and multiple pairs of socks over the past few years.

l.   Wash your hands before and after every physical exam

General Surgery

a.   Sleep is at a premium. You'll be rounding at six or six thirty in the morning., which means that you'll need to get up at five or five thirty. You'll need to go to bed earlier to make it through this rotation. Most places do not serve coffee at this time, so make your own or wait until later.

b.   Rounding is in a team, and can initially be overwhelming. If you have some free time later in the day, try to go through the charts to get to know your patients.

c.   The OR's generally start at seven thirty or eight in the morning. Make sure you're well hydrated and have eaten breakfast. I also require a coffee. The OR's can be several hours long and as a medical student, your job will be retracting to expose the surgical field (looks like water skiing) and cutting sutures. You may have an opportunity to close the skin. Wear comfortable shoes and if you need them, wear compression stockings.

d.   While in the OR, it's traditional for the surgeon or upper-year residents to quiz the medical student. Read the case list the night before to get an idea of what topics might be asked of you.

e.   Carry portable food with you. The time you'll have available to eat is limited. Granola bars, yogurt in tubes, nuts, and cans of tomato juice are good emergency energy sources. If you can make it to the cafeteria, many clerks swear by the soothing properties of chocolate milk.

f.   Ask questions about what you see. It's a privilege to be in an OR, so make the best of this amazing opportunity.

g.   Always meet your patients before you go into an OR with them. You'll often get to do a history and physical before you begin. Not only is this a common courtesy, but you should also use this chance to better understand what you're about to see.

h.   If you want more hands-on experiences, go to the smaller, shorter surgeries. These "entry-level" surgeries such as hernia repairs, appendectomies, and lumpectomies may give you more of an opportunity to participate.

i.   Always stay to help with the transfer of the patient off the OR table onto the stretcher. Be nice, and ask if you can help by bringing in the warm blankets or moving the stretcher to recovery. Write an OR note with help if you need it. Take a stab at post-op orders and review them with the resident.

j.   Don't forget your friends. The amount of time spent in the hospital during general surgery, plus the need to maximize your time for sleeping and studying, can wear you down. Make a point of spending some time doing something that's not related to surgery.

k.   If you get a needle stick, report it. You'll sleep better if you take care of yourself.

l.   Ask a resident to teach you how to tie a one-handed surgical knot, both overhand and underhand. You'll impress your staff and amaze your friends.

Family Medicine

a.   Family medicine offers the most variety of all the specialties. If you have a particular interest, for example *family obstetrics* or *family geriatrics*, see if you can work with a family doctor who's involved in that area of care.

b. If you get the chance, work with a rural family doctor. This will really give you a chance to see the breadth of this field of medicine. You'll likely get to work in a clinic, deliver babies, assist in the O.R., and work in the emergency department.

c. Work on developing an approach to a number of common family medicine problems such as hypertension, diabetes, back pain, fever, depression, paediatric milestones, fatigue, sexually transmitted diseases, asthma, and headache.

d. Be prepared to incorporate general health screening into your interviews, such as vaccinations, seatbelt and helmet use, and mammography.

e. Family practice can be very busy and often people have waited long past their appointment time until they're seen. If someone is venting their frustration to you, sympathize with the patient without placing blame on anyone.

f. If you have the opportunity to see the same patient in a follow-up visit, go for it. This is what family medicine is about—continuity of care. Find out what happened to your patient from one week to another.

Psychiatry

a. This rotation is different from most others in that you're not constantly charging around the hospital. You'll grow accustomed to sitting for extended periods of time.

b. Some people find this rotation overwhelming as it brings up certain feelings from their own past, especially if they themselves or a family member has suffered from a mental illness. If you're having difficulties, speak to a staff about it sooner rather than later

c. Find a way to organize your interview. Most admission interviews take about an hour to do, after which you can often narrow down your diagnosis. It can be a challenge at first to find out the information without getting too off-topic.

d. If you're threatened or feel in danger, get out. Make sure the room is set up so that the patient is not between you and the door.

e. It's sometimes hard to remember the details of a one-hour interview later on, so sometimes you'll have to take notes. Find a way to get the essential information recorded (e.g., ages, family members, dates.) that you're unlikely to remember without spending the entire time with your head bent over your paper. It's a delicate balance.

Internal Medicine

a. Mornings in internal medicine usually start out with a series of rounding cycles. First, you should round on your own patients and write a note on each. Keep track of specific questions and issues. Next, you'll usually round with your senior resident. Keep a set of X-ray and physiotherapy forms in your pocket so you can fill them out as you go. After this, you may or may not round with your staff. This series of rounding can sometimes take all morning. Your afternoons are likely to be spent organizing treatment plans, discharging patients, or following up on results.

b. Internal medicine is usually divided into teams, with each team lead by a senior resident under a staff person, each responsible for a certain group of patients. When you're on call, you're often on call as a team, covering the floors and the ER. Because there are so many people working at the same time seeing such a huge volume of patients, make sure you communicate what's going on with the people you're seeing with the senior or another resident.

c. You need to be organized in internal medicine. You'll likely be given a few patients of your own that you're responsible for rounding on each day. Find a system that allows you to track their vitals, lab results, and test reports so that you can follow up each day on their progress.

d. See as many patients as you can in the ER. Going to see these consults will give you a first hand look at how various illnesses present. You'll likely be given enough time to do a thorough history and examination, and look at initial tests such as X-rays and EKGs. If you end up admitting a patient through the ER, follow their care while in hospital.

e.   There's a tonne of paperwork in internal medicine, often because many of the patients are chronically ill and require various levels of care after being discharged. It's up to the team to find placements in long-term care facilities, nursing homes, or registering patients in rehabilitation or physio programs.

The On-Call Kit

1.   New socks and fresh knickers. Put these on in the morning and you will feel 100% fresher.

2.   Toothpaste, toothbrush, deodorant, and face wipes (use when you lie down and get up to round. If you do not sleep at all, try to use these before you start rounding again – it'll help wake you up).

3.   Small tube of hand lotion and lip balm. It's very dry in hospitals, and it's hard to remember to drink enough. Keep your hands moisturized to protect them from cracking, as cracked skin is a route for infection if you're accidentally splashed with body fluids. Use a tube of lip balm and not a jar; you don't want to put your fingers into it after touching a doorknob or a chart in a hospital.

4.   Food: I basically live off granola bars when I'm on call. They're compact, can be eaten quickly, and fit in your lab coat pocket. I also usually bring some yogurt (especially if there's a fridge), cans of tomato juice (makes sure I get my vegetables), and some fruit that will not get squished (apples and oranges, good; kiwis and bananas, bad). Most hospitals have coffee shops or restaurants, but they're rarely open twenty-four hours a day. Some of them close as early as 6:00 p.m. and are not open at all on weekends. It's not uncommon for you to have your first chance to eat something after everything has shut down, so you need to plan for this and have something available to you.

5. A bottle of water and a couple cans of pop. Again, dehydration is the enemy. A big glass of cool water or fizzy pop can be just the thing to re-energize you at four in the morning.

6. A t-shirt to wear underneath your scrubs. Most hospitals are quite cold, and many people on call start to feel really cold at about three or four in the morning. You cannot wear a t-shirt on top of your scrubs in many areas of the hospital (near the operating room, for example), so just get used to wearing them underneath. Hospital garb is also not known for its downy softness, so avoid body-chap and wear a t-shirt.

7. Notebook: get a small one that has pages you can tear out and fits in the pocket of your scrubs. Write down pass codes, your Sr.'s pager number, and other important numbers on the first page. Also use this to keep notes on patients

8. Pens, pens, pens!

9. Peripheral brain.

10. Stethoscope.

11. Comfy shoes. The first time I was on call, I fell asleep with my running shoes on so I wouldn't have to work to get my shoes on if I was paged in an emergency (essentially sleeping with my boots on). The next day, my feet hurt and stank. I now have a pair of very comfortable slip-on shoes that I can easily slide on and off. Find a good pair of comfortable shoes that you don't need to tie but will stay on your feet if you're running. Don't get shoes with holes (air vents) in them; if you're splashed with body fluids while delivering a baby or in the operating room, your socks will be soaked. Make sure they're made of a material that can be easily wiped off if something does spill on them.

12. Gum, otherwise known as the clerk's toothbrush. You and your patients will feel much better at three in the morning if you can chew a piece of minty gum. You'll also feel more confident interacting with your colleagues the following morning, assuming you had no time to brush. Remember that *SuperClerk* has worked all night but comes off looking as fresh as a daisy.

Doc Talk

Tips for on call:
Don't be scared, your resident is there. The first time I was on call, I was really nervous, and it's wonderful to have your PGY1 there.
It's cold in the call room. In some rooms you can crank up the heat, but in others you'll have to lug out some blankets.

—*Midori Yamamoto, 4th year Medical Student*

Peripheral Brain (PDA)

During my clerkship, and also while I interned, there were three things that I found I used almost every day. In order of importance, they are:

1. Pens. As a physician, your pen is your sword. Your notes set the stage and your orders are the actors. You'll use your pen more than any other tool. Keep many, many pens available at all times and do not be caught without one. There's a great pen cycle by which pens are lost and pens are found, but it's more professional to just always have one with you.

2. Your stethoscope. This tool is used in almost every discipline of medicine, and can assess the heart, the lungs, and the bowels, find evidence of sclerosis in large arteries, can be used to check reflexes, and often can distract and amuse young children. If you're ever asked to assess a patient, bring your stethoscope. It's probably the only piece of medical equipment actually worth buying as a medical student. I was silly enough to buy an otoscope as a medical student, an instrument principally used to look in ears. As a resident in ob-gyn, this $500 investment is mostly used to amuse my family by telling them how much wax is in their ears.

3. Your PDA or peripheral brain. If you're going to spend money on something technological, I'd highly recommend a PDA. There are a number of searchable medical texts available for PDAs, which will make your life all the easier in a number of clinical scenarios. I'd also recommend that you get a good drug program for when you're writing orders and need to look up dosages.

Many PDAs have enough memory to save a Power Point presentation, so if you need to present at rounds (which you will) you don't have to carry a laptop around all day. Get a PDA, make sure you're comfortable using it, and keep it charged. Personally, my peripheral brain also has a cell phone in it, which is invaluable when I'm on home-call and need to return a page. It's my medical reference, drug reference, calendar, document holder, rolodex, and phone. I can't tell you how many times I was glad I had it when I was on call as an intern.

Studying During Clerkship

*"The hardest conviction to get into the mind of the beginner is that the education
upon which she is engaged is not a college course,
not a medical course, but a life course."*
—*Sir William Osler*

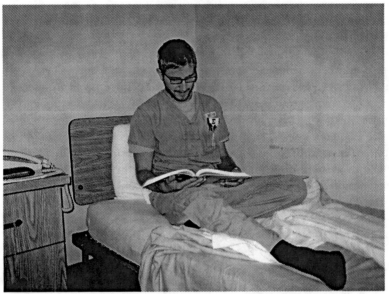

A clinical clerk catches up on some reading while on call

There are a number of responsibilities during clerkship. There
will be responsibilities to your team, your patients, and to your
learning. Sometimes it will seem like there aren't enough hours in a
day, especially when your sleep schedule is thrown off by being on
call. You'll be presented with huge amounts of information and things
will be happening quickly. You'll see a resident make a decision and
not know why, you'll see clinical findings you don't understand, and
you'll be presented with a patient and you won't know where to start.
In such a hectic environment, how will you keep up with patients?
How will you find the time and the peace to get through that
textbook and memorize its contents?

First of all, you'll probably be getting a lot more out of your
patient encounters than out of reading a textbook. Medicine is
practiced with your five senses (okay, doctors don't taste their

patients' urine anymore, so I guess it's just four senses), so your textbook at this point is a supplement to your knowledge to fuel your true doctoring skills. You need to know this textbook information so you can put it into context, but in the end, it's being able to apply it to real situations that matters; because there are tests, and then there are *tests*. Tests are written at the end of a rotation and you get a grade on them, *tests* happen at four in the morning with a crashing patient when you're the first one on the scene. You cannot cram for tests anymore. You actually need to know what's going on and retain it, so you know what to do when the real *test* comes.

You need to integrate your learning. It's the only way to keep up with your patients, get through the core material for the rotation, and retain the information for when you need it most. This essentially comes down to reading around your patients. When you see someone in the ER, on the ward, or a patient is assigned to you, write down the name of their clinical condition and the issues surrounding it. Those topics are your reading assignments for that night. If you have the opportunity to read about it during the day, even better. In fact, I found that seeing a patient, reading about them, and then re-visiting them to be very reinforcing. If you have a PDA with a good database, you can easily look up medical information without disrupting the flow of a clinic. If you have easy access to a computer, you can get on the Internet to learn more while at work. Ask your resident about the condition. If they like to teach, your resident may show you an "approach" to the condition, which is a way of breaking something down into smaller parts, be it treatment plans, a diagnostic work-up, aetiology, outcomes, or a differential diagnosis. It's basically a way of organizing large amounts of information into logical patterns to help you understand and remember it.

If you continue to read around your patients for the duration of your rotation, chances are that you'll have covered the majority of the core material needed for the exit exam. If there are topics that you've missed because you haven't had a patient encounter that prompted the reading, go back at the end of the rotation and read about those.

The key to reading around your patients is learning to ask yourself the right questions. For example, imagine you have a patient with pancreatitis. You might ask yourself, what causes pancreatitis? How does it present clinically? What tests can you order to figure out if it's pancreatitis or not? What else could it be? Who gets pancreatitis? What are the major concerns in the long-term and in the short-term? Why are people worried about this patient's fluid balance? The patient asked if this will happen again - will it? How long will it take for him to get better? It's one thing to read about how to find the JVP (an indicator of fluid status), but it's something totally different to actually perform this physical exam on a patient and use it to help you make a clinical decision.

You'll sometimes be prompted by residents or staff about what issues are important. Read about these, and if you have a chance, follow up with the person who asked you the question. Having an active conversation about a real patient with someone experienced in the field will help you remember things much more easily. If you're going to a clinic or assisting the OR, find out what the clinic is for or find the OR list the day before. This will allow you to read about the topic ahead of time and you'll get a lot more from your patient encounters.

I've found that these skills served me well both as a student and as a resident. Figuring out what to read and how to apply that information is a skill that will improve over time. Having real patients in need of your care is an extremely motivating reason to keep up with the knowledge base!

Doc Talk

Now that I'm into my first year of clinical work, I feel tired all the time. I never felt this way before because I was always able to catch up on sleep on weekends. Doing this long-term really is difficult. I guess you learn about yourself, and you don't know until you put yourself though it what type of career you want.

—Midori Yamamoto, 4th year medical student

The reality of medicine: Everyone around you is going down the same road. So day-to-day it doesn't seem so crazy. If you take a step back and compare it to your friends who are not in medicine, it might make you ask yourself what the hell you're doing, but it doesn't seem so weird that you have crazy hours and all those years in school.

—Dr. Rickesh Sood, 2nd year family medicine resident

CHAPTER 12: THINKING ABOUT RESIDENCY

Choosing Your Specialty

HOW do you go about choosing what you want to do after you graduate from medical school? Whether you've taken a three- or four-year program, many clerks still feel like there's not enough time to choose a residency program. People often start out in medical school visualizing themselves as one type of doctor, and then end up doing something completely different. Only 11% of doctors ended up in the area of speciality they imagined for themselves at the start of medical school. Compare that to the 53% who chose their area of speciality during clerkship *(National Physician Survey-Resident Questionnaires, 2004)*.

When I started medical school, the two areas of medicine that I'd had previous exposure with were endocrinology and obstetrics and gynaecology. I'd worked on research projects with physicians in both these areas while in university. Initially, I visualized myself as a family doctor or paediatrician because I wanted to participate in preventative medicine and I was worried about doing a lot of call. I was also pretty sure that I didn't want to do any type of surgery. I soon decided that I had been too hasty to rule out anything that involves working in the OR, so I did an elective in otolaryngology. Although I wasn't drawn to the topic, I discovered that I love being in the OR, and really liked the split between OR time and clinic time. I was encouraged to try ob-gyn, and I found it was the perfect balance between medicine, surgery, and preventative care.

So, I was back where I started. During this time I also seriously considered both general surgery and psychiatry, and although I entered each clerkship rotation with an open mind, I realized that I didn't enjoy some rotations as much I thought I would. When I applied for residency, I was certain of my decision and I applied exclusively for ob-gyn positions.

So, how can you go about deciding what you want to do in residency?

1. Consider your educational background. If you've done research in a certain field of study, as either an undergraduate or graduate student, you most probably have an innate interest in that area. You may have decided to apply to medical school with the intention of being a doctor and researcher or are now discovering the clinical implications of your area of expertise. You might also find yourself more comfortable and confident in this area of medicine because of your extensive exposure to it from a research or academic perspective. Your research in this area will also be a great asset to your residency application. The only danger here is the development of specialty tunnel-vision, where you're certain about what you want to do and don't attempt to explore any other areas of medicine.

2. Consider your personal experience. Maybe you or a family member has experienced an illness that drove you to pursue medicine. You may deeply sympathize with patients who also suffer from similar conditions and find you have a great sense of vocation towards this area. I know that my personal experience in rural Mexico gave me a sense of vocation towards international health, and I felt ob-gyn provided opportunities to participate in international health. As with considering your educational background, it's still important to explore other areas to prevent tunnel-vision.

3. You had a great rotation. Many people find that there's an area of medicine that they enjoy and where they feel at home. If you're having a great time and loving the patient interactions, you're having in a certain rotation, chances are you'll continue to do so. To get a better idea of the scope of the field, try attending a conference and take electives with preceptors at different sites.

4. You found a mentor. There may be a staff person who you feel you connect with who encourages you to apply to their area of

specialty. Perhaps you feel that you have a similar personality and can easily visualise yourself doing the same thing. The caveat here is to make sure that you actually like the discipline for what it is, not just because someone you admire is in it.

5. Career days. You may have the chance to attend career days or career lunches, where doctors from different specialties talk about what they do. This can be a good door-opener, especially for some of the areas of medicine that do not get a lot of exposure during clerkship such as community medicine, ophthalmology, or palliative care.

6. Start with something broad. Try something that can expose you to a wide range of topics like a first elective or during your pre-clinical years at medical school. Rural family medicine is a good starter because many rural family physicians work shifts in the ER, run a family clinic, deliver babies, and assist in the operating room. This will give you a taste of many areas of medicine in one elective. Electives in urban family medicine or ER can also provide an experience with a wide variety of patient types.

7. Medical or surgical? This is often the first question that needs to be answered. Specialties that require quite a bit of technical skill, or *hand specialties* include general surgery, orthopaedic surgery, neurosurgery, otolaryngology, urology, plastic surgery, and cardiac surgery. Medical specialties, or *head specialties*, include internal medicine, radiology, pathology, medical genetics, paediatrics, and psychiatry. Some specialties lean heavily to the *hand* side or the *head* side, whereas others offer more of a balance, such as obstetrics and gynaecology, anaesthesia, and emergency medicine. How would you prefer to spend your day?

8. Specialist or generalist? This tends to be divided between knowing a lot about a small area of medicine or a little about everything. Do you like to dive deeply into something, or would you prefer to be a jack-of-all-trades?

9. Lifestyle. This is an important consideration, and it's taking on an ever increasing role in the career decision-making process of graduating medical students. What else do you want out of life? How willing are you to have your home life disrupted to take care of patients? Being on call from home lets you stay at home but

prevents you from going away for the weekend. You may have to cancel plans at the last minute or leave important events. Being on call in the hospital means missing time with your family and sleepless nights. Different areas of medicine give you different levels of control over your hours. Doctors in the same field of medicine have a variety of ways of dividing up the call schedule to ensure that their patients always have access to a physician. This often depends on practice group size, services offered, and size of the community being serviced.

For example, in obstetrics and gynaecology, doctors working in a large centre are on call only a few times per month, but the call is extremely busy, and sleep is a rarity. In more rural areas with only two or three ob-gyns, they're on call every second or third day, but may only do one or two deliveries each day.

I'm only using this to illustrate that there are many possibilities within every discipline, but some will inevitably have more call than others. Endocrinologists are rarely called in the middle of the night because of an emergency, whereas a general surgeon can count on it. You'll have to make sacrifices to your career, your life outside of medicine, or both. What balance are you happy with? What other responsibilities do you have? What are you willing to give up? How do the people who love you feel about you cancelling plans or not coming home when expected? How do you feel about spending at least a few nights of every month in the hospital for the rest of your career? How do you feel about not ever having a regular sleep schedule again? Are you a morning person? A night person? Are you a grump to live with if you've under-slept? Are you willing to make less money if it means you have more control over your schedule? Are you okay with having a pager wake you and your spouse up in the middle of the night? Are you willing to spend five years in a gruelling residency program if it means that you'll have more control over your life after you finish? What other goals and dreams do you have? Are you defined by your doctor-hood, or does something else define you? How well do you manage stress? Think about these questions, talk to staff in the field, and find out what your life, not just your career, might be like.

10. Options for career growth and change. Deciding to become a doctor is usually a life-long career decision. But how much

flexibility is there in your field of choice as you go through different stages of your life? When you have kids? When you're aging? When you have ample free time? What fellowships, academic opportunities, and areas of focus are available to you as you progress through your life stages? Can your career grow and change with you? What can you do with your education if you're tired of your pager going off every night?

11. How do you feel at the end of the day? I think this is a very important question. Life doesn't stop when you leave your hospital or clinic for the night. Are you still your best self? Are you happy? Are you stressed out, fatigued, or sad? I loved my general surgery rotation, but only while I was in the hospital. I found that at the end of the day I had nothing left to give. I stopped participating in my extracurricular activities and started wearing jogging pants around the house way too often. All I wanted to do was sleep and eat. I decided not to pursue this career because of who I was while I wasn't doing it. I felt the same way about family medicine, even though the hours and stress levels were much less! However, I came home excited, energized, and looking forward to the next day in obstetrics and gynaecology. This was a huge factor in my career decision.

12. Is the residency worth it? Specialist residencies are five years in length, a significant period of time when someone else will be in charge of your schedule. You'll be paid relatively little, and you'll be working exceptionally hard. Do you need this to get what you want out of medicine? Is putting in the five years worth it to you? Or could you get what you want out of medicine through a two-year family residency and perhaps a short fellowship (e.g., family anaesthesia, family obstetrics, family palliative, family emergency)?

Doc Talk

I didn't know I wanted to do family medicine in the beginning. I think many of us go through a bit of a journey in medical school about what you want to do. I remember people saying I had to pick between surgery and medicine, and between acute or chronic medicine. Part of taking my year off to do my masters was to think about what I wanted to do and where I wanted to go. I thought that Mac was so quick, and you really have to feel decisive. I think that's really difficult in a three-year medical school. Probably also in a four-year medical school. I think you have to get yourself out of that academic environment. You're taught in medical school by specialists, not by family doctors, and so you don't really get a family medicine point of view.

–Dr. Rickesh Sood, 2nd year family medicine resident

It shocked me what I did and didn't like. I thought I would like family medicine but I hated it; the pressure that's on family doctors is awful. I thought I would hate surgery and anaesthesia, but I loved them.

–Dr. Jennifer Graham, 1st year paediatrics resident

This is a hard decision; you might already have a gut feeling about what you want to end up doing. Just make sure that you explore your options, think about your life outside medicine, and be true to yourself. This is like deciding to become a doctor in the first place. Don't let anyone bully you into a specialty because they feel it's more prestigious or you'll be happier. This is a decision you have to make for yourself based on your personality and career and life goals.

Medical Electives

Doc Talk

You need to surround yourself with doctors who are the type of doctor you want to be. If you work with someone who's always swearing and being annoyed by patients, you'll often end up modeling that behaviour. I think that you're a product of your environment and your mentors. But if you work with someone who has qualities that you admire, you'll probably learn to treat patients the way they do. So do electives with people you want to be like.

–Christopher McCrossin, 4th year medical student

All medical programs allow you to take elective time, meaning that you get to plan an educational experience in the field and location of your choice. Some schools group all of this time together in the last year of medical school, whereas others spread it throughout the clerkship years. There are many ways to use this time, but most people use it as a chance to plan for residency in one way or another. Most people spend two to four weeks at a specific elective, as this gives you enough time to get to know the people you're working with and explore an area of interest without spending all of your time in one place.

Apply for electives early. If you're applying for an elective at another university, you often need to have the paperwork in place months in advance. Paperwork for international electives are often required at least six months in advance. You often need to go through the electives office at the university you're applying to, and they'll check for availability of electives in your area of interest. If you know of a preceptor that you specifically want to work with, you should contact them directly first. If you're hoping to work with a physician who's associated with a university, you'll usually be charged a fee to apply. I think this is generally a money grab, as each medical school sends out and accepts students from other medical schools where they're all paying tuition already.

If you're going away for an elective, you'll need to find a place to stay. Many people stay with family and friends if they know someone in the area, while others can sometimes get a decent rate at a bed and breakfast for a month. In the summer you can sometimes find sublets in university areas. Certain hospitals and some rural elective programs may provide an apartment or living space in the hospital. Overall, when the application fees, transportation, and extra living expenses add up (sometimes you'll find yourself paying rent for two apartments at once!) electives can be quite expensive. This is definitely a mandatory expense, especially if you want to get into a specific program. Take this into consideration when you're working out your budget for medical school.

Many clerks are forced into booking electives before they've really experienced most areas of medicine. And because electives often set the stage for residency, they need to make decisions based on very little real information. You will often be able to choose in what order you complete your clerkship rotations, and there's a certain strategy to picking the best order. For example, imagine you're fairly certain that you want to do paediatrics. You wouldn't want this to be your first rotation because you're still becoming comfortable with the hospital and seeing patients every day, finding out how things work, how to order X-rays, and building up your confidence. Regardless on what rotation people start, during their first rotation clerks have less confidence, among other things. They're just starting to learn how to do this doctoring thing, because it really is just the first few days on the job. Clerks can show that they're hard-working during their very first rotation, but it's much harder to show poise under pressure, awesome history, physical skills, and general coolness.

At the same time, you don't want to put paediatrics right at the end. If you do that you'll miss your chance to discover early on whether or not you actually like it. It's also advisable to have completed your core rotation in an area before you go off and do electives in it. This is vital if you are to impress your supervisors during your electives.

If you have one choice that you're really considering, I'd suggest making it your second or third rotation. If you have two choices that you're considering, make one your second rotation and one your third. This should give you enough time to warm up to becoming a good clerk, as well as enough time to set up electives and change your mind if necessary.

How Can I Use My Elective Time?

1) Exploration elective: The goal of this type of elective is to explore career options or residency locations in greater depth. Did you enjoy general surgery the first time around, only to be left wondering if it was the excitement of a new rotation that pulled you in, or if it really is your dream career? Are you interested in family medicine but don't know if you fit in with the staff at a certain university?
Can't decide between internal medicine and paediatrics?

You can use your electives to answer some of these questions. Many people already have some idea of what specialty they're interested in and just want to make sure. Others love two distinct areas of medicine and use some elective time to help make this decision. It's probably a good idea to try at least a few areas of medicine as electives, so you don't box yourself into a career too quickly. I've heard people say, "I love obstetrics and gynaecology, but I've already booked all my electives and have a research project in ENT. If I'd tried this earlier I probably would have wanted to do it." So use a couple of weeks to try stuff out! The goals of an exploration elective often overlap with an *interview elective*.

2) Interview elective: Doing an elective at a specific university and program gives the staff a chance to really get to know you. Most people use the majority of their elective time on *interview electives*. If you're convinced that psychiatry at Queen's is the program you really want to be in, then you should definitely do an elective there, preferably with either the director of the program or someone who's on the resident selection committee. This gives you a chance to impress your preceptor, see how well you fit in, and hopefully get a positive letter of reference outlining how you would make a great member of their team. You need to be "on" throughout this elective, getting to know people, doing as much call as you're able to, and reading around cases at night. You need to be your best self to all members of the team, including nursing staff, administrative personnel, other residents, medical students, and of course, the staff. It's pretty common for medical students to ask for a letter of recommendation at the end of an elective. Most people make their interview electives a little longer than an exploration elective so that they can really become part of the team. For example, if you're just considering palliative care because you heard someone else really enjoyed it, you might use a smaller amount of your time than if you were certain you wanted to be a neurologist and were trying to impress a residency director.

It's sometimes difficult to know how to space out your time if you're certain of a specialty but not a location. If you already know what you want to do, I'd suggest spreading your time as evenly as possible across the locations. This will give you the best chance of getting to know the programs as much as possible, without putting all your eggs in one basket.

3) Reading elective: Reading electives generally involves in-depth reading surrounding an area of interest. You usually need to prepare a summary of what you've learned or have an oral exam with your preceptor to prove you did the work. Generally, I'd think the only reason you'd want to do a reading elective is if you need to fill in elective time while traveling for CaRMS interview. A clinical or research elective is generally a much better use of your time.

4) Research elective: There are two types of research elective. The first is working on research for a previous or concurrent degree while getting credit for it at medical school. The second is to do research in an area of interest. Doing medical research demonstrates your intent to learn more about an area of specialty and is a good way to get to know staff people in your field of interest. You should approach staff people and find out who's doing a project that they need some help with. If you're lucky you'll be able to publish or present your findings. These are all very good things when applying to residency.

5) International elective: If you have the time and the money to do this, go. You'll never regret taking time during medical school to travel and learn. I spent a month in the Royal Kingdom of Tonga working with Tongan physicians. I had an amazing time and learned a lot about cultural determinants of health and international medicine. International electives can take place in developing countries like Tonga or Zimbabwe, or at well-known institutions like the London School of Hygiene and Tropical Medicine.

Before you go, make sure the institution that's accepting you is aware of your level of training and is able to provide proper supervision of your activities. You're not there to "practice" on people from other countries! Look into and be aware of cultural differences and language barriers that could affect your elective. If the languages you're fluent in are not widely spoken, is there someone who can act as an interpreter? This is important because interacting with patients without understanding them can significantly hinder your ability to learn from the experience. Make sure you research the safety of the elective. You would want to know if there was political instability, if you needed certain vaccinations, if you would have access to medications in case of a needle stick from a high risk HIV patient, and other questions relevant to the area visited. If you're travelling to a developing country, find out beforehand if there are certain supplies that are most in need by the hospital and find out if they would be interested in a donation. Ask what's needed before bringing random donations. While in Tonga, I saw piles of orthopaedic equipment gathering dust in a corner because there was no orthopaedic surgeon, and surgical soap that was unused because it came without the equipment that allowed it to be dispensed in a sterile fashion.

When traveling abroad, find out what paperwork is needed to transport drugs into the country before you go to avoid loosing your donation at the border. I highly recommend an international elective—just make sure you educate yourself before you go.

6) Last chance elective: People sometimes take an elective after the match is completed in an area where they're just not comfortable. It's your last chance to do some clinical learning as a student before they throw you out on the wards as a first-year resident. Many people who feel this way choose to do something they've had little experience in. Ophthalmology or dermatology are good examples. Others want to brush up generally and do something like family medicine or internal medicine.

7) The Post-CaRMS fun-time elective: Some schools have elective time available after the match. This can be extremely freeing because at this point you're no longer trying to impress anyone, and you can essentially do whatever piques your interest. If this is not a *last chance elective*, you can do something you've always wanted to but never got around to, like hypnotherapy, an elective in your home town, traveling to a city you've always wanted to visit, or working with a doctor who does house calls.

CaRMS or The Match

Shortly after you enter medical school, people will start talking about residency. It's actually amazing how quickly your perception can change from, "Thank goodness I got into medical school - now all I have to do is study hard and I'll be a doctor," to, "Wow. - I'd better start thinking about what type of doctor I want to be, set up appropriate electives, and do research, or I won't match."

The match, or CaRMS (the Canadian Resident Matching Service) is an application process that all graduating medical students must go through to achieve a residency position. You cannot practice medicine in Canada without completing a residency, even though you have an M.D. Residency is between two and six years in length, and during this time you're providing service at the same time as getting an education.

This process is reminiscent of applying to medical school, as you're again asked to write a letter of intent, provide your medical school and sometimes undergraduate transcripts, and get letters of recommendation. The focus is no longer on why you're suited for medicine in general, but why you're suited to become a certain type of physician. This is followed by a cross-Canada adventure of interviewing at a number of universities.

Each program makes a list of applying candidates, ranking them from first to last based on who they'd most like in their program. At the same time, you'll make a list of your own, ranking the programs in order of preference, also first to last. A computer program analyses the two lists and matches your highest choice to a program that also ranked you highly. It sounds quite confusing, but it's actually quite fair. Basically, you'll get the spot you most prefer if there's room for you. The best strategy is to order your list in the honest order of your preference, rank every school that you would be willing to go to, and do not rank a program you would not attend if you were given the spot. When you apply through CaRMS, you must also sign a contract stating that you will attend whichever school you are matched to.

If you're graduating from a Canadian medical school the year you're applying through CaRMS, you are automatically eligible for the first iteration of the match. This means that when you apply, all the residency spots are available to you. If you go unmatched, you're only able to apply to the leftover spots in the second iteration. These are positions that were not able to find a suitable candidate in the first iteration.

The application process for the match starts the August before you graduate, and interviews are generally held in January and February. It's hard, but you should try to start filling out your application early. I was trying to write my application letters the same time I was doing my internal medicine clerkship rotation. You need to write a letter of intent for each school and each program you're applying to, and provide letters of reference for each program you're applying to. This means, for example, that if you're applying to both psychiatry and family medicine, you need references that are specific to those programs. You may find that you need different references for different schools. One family medicine program might want a reference specifically from one of their staff, whereas another might want a reference that shows your interest in rural practice. Putting this all together is time consuming and you'll find yourself fretting over organizing it meticulously. In the end, most people are invited for interviews at most places.

Interviewing can be quite expensive, requiring multiple plane tickets, hotel stays, dining out, and often a new suit or two. Many people try to stay with relatives, and there's a system in place for medical students to host interviewees who need a place to sleep. You'll probably start seeing some familiar people along the way as you travel from coast to coast. It can be a great way to have a whirlwind tour of Canadian capital cities! Take the time to prepare for your interview. It's amazing how much time you'll spend preparing, writing, and editing your letters of intent, and how little you can spend preparing for the actual interview. Go through the same type of questions that you used to prepare for your medical school interview. You'll find at this point that you'll have actual clinical situations to draw upon to make your points. Most interviews ask how you've handled a situation in the past, your experience and understanding of ethical principles in medicine, and your understanding of the discipline. Usually you're not required to demonstrate actual knowledge in an area (e.g., "Describe the clinical presentation of hypothyroidism"), but I've heard of it happening. Personally, I think you'll probably get more out of going over your clinical experiences, thinking about what made you choose that discipline, and what big-picture lessons you've learned in medicine.

Here's an example of a question I was asked: "Tell me about a time that you made a mistake communicating while you were a medical student."

Answer: "When I was a clerk, there was a patient who had incompletely miscarried and needed a D and C. The staff went with me to get consent for the procedure. I explained what they did, and there was a box at the bottom of the form to give consent for blood products. The patient was scared and had been crying, and asked about the box. I told her that it was to give permission for blood products if she needed them, but she looked so scared that I said, 'But the probability of that is like one in a million.' The staff cut in and said the probability is actually about one in one hundred, and he continued to explain the form to her. I felt awful. I realized that my need to make her feel better, because she looked so scared, was overriding her right to accurate information. I've never made that mistake again."

During your interview, there are some illegal questions. They're not allowed to ask about your marital status, children, desire for children (are you planning on getting pregnant during residency?), what other programs you're applying to, or where you'll rank their program for the match. You can bring up these topics yourself if you want, but they're not allowed to ask specifically about them.

Match day is usually in March. Match day is usually extremely emotional; people are excited, relieved, disappointed, or scared. It often means moving to a new city, and many people are hit with the sudden realization that they really are going to be a surgeon, a family doctor, or a dermatologist. I remember going out with some friends a few weeks after the match and realizing that between the ten of us we could staff a small hospital; we had all the principle disciplines represented.

You can read more about the process of the match at the official website, http://www.carms.ca

Match Strategies

You need to first decide on your priority: location, program, or matching with someone else (a *couple's match* is available for people who want to end up in the same location. Often people do find the love of their life in medical school!).

Also, keep in mind that there's no such thing as a shoe-in. It's in a program director's best interest to attract as many people to their program as possible, and have medical students rank their program highly. A program director who says something along the lines of, "I wouldn't worry about the match if I were you," or, "The interview is only a formality," is not necessarily speaking the truth. It's not over until match day, baby.

If the program is your most important consideration, apply to every single school that offers that program in the country. There's no penalty for applying to multiple schools, and interviewers are not allowed to ask you what other programs you're applying to. For example, if you're applying to orthopaedic surgery, apply to every program in the country.

Next, if you're thinking of backing up with a second program, back up with programs that are the same length in years, preferably in the same school or at least the same province. This is for funding purposes. Each spot has a certain number of years of funding associated with it, and it's easier to switch out of something if the funding is in place. For example, switching from orthopaedics to general surgery both at University of Toronto (same number of years, same school) is logistically easiest, whereas switching form family medicine at Queen's to radiology at UBC would be logistically most difficult (you only have two years of funding with family and you need five years of funding for radiology; it's also an inter-provincial move).

Many people back up with family medicine. Please only do this if you really think you'll be happy as a family physician. Because of the way that the funding structure runs, switching out of family can be hit or miss.

If location is most important, rank every discipline you would be happy with at your favourite location, followed by locations nearby or in the same province. Remember that if you're planning on attempting to transfer later, it's easier to do so within the same province. Of course, you'll likely have a discipline that you would prefer, and there is usually a combination of preference of location and discipline.

In a *couple's match*, you rank together combinations of locations and programs. The couple's match is much more competitive in terms of your likelihood of getting your first choice, since both programs have to accept both people for a match to be made.

The general rule for the match is to be honest about what will make you happiest. Pay no attention to any promises made prior to match day by program directors. Rank your favourite program first even if you think it's a long shot. Never rank a program that you would not attend. If you're thinking about attempting a transfer as a back-up plan, make sure that you'd honestly be happy in that program, either the discipline or the location, as transfers are not always possible.

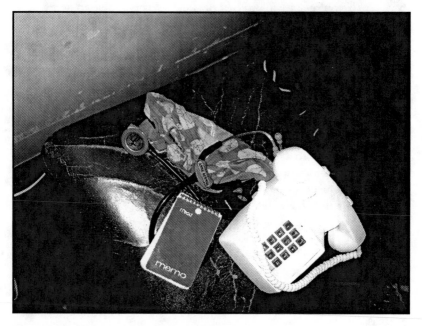

Being on call, your gear near the phone

The Match for International Medical Graduates

If you're a Canadian citizen or permanent resident and you've completed your medical school abroad, you're eligible for the match if you've passed the MCCEE and have not yet undergone any residency training. If you apply to residency positions in Quebec or Manitoba, you apply in direct competition to Canadian graduates and have no return of service obligations. Newfoundland, Nova Scotia, Ontario, and British Columbia will allow to you to apply in *parallel*, meaning there are a certain number of spots specifically for internationally trained medical graduates, and you will also have a return of service obligation. Saskatchewan and Alberta do not offer spots in the first iteration to international medical graduates.

What If I Don't Match?

There's a small possibility that you'll fail to match to any program. This is most often caused by applying only to extremely competitive disciplines (dermatology, ENT, plastics). The lack of a match can also be caused by applying to less programs than you should. If you fail to match you're automatically entered into the second iteration of the match. This means that you're eligible to compete for the residency programs that have not yet found a resident to fill their spot. The problem with this is that it's much less likely that you'll find a position in the specialty area that you were originally interested in, and historically the majority of these spots have been family medicine.

The second iteration requires that you start your application all over again, and you need a new letter of intent and new letters of recommendation. Overall, the process is generally stressful. Some people find an area of specialty that's similar to their original area of application. They may have applied to ENT, for example (which is very competitive), and not matched. There may be a spot available in general surgery, and after being accepted to this position there might (if they're very lucky) be an opportunity to switch into ENT at a later date. You should realise, though, that all programs are aware that the applicants in the second iteration are thinking of ways to get back into their first choice program. People who match in the second iteration start residency on July 1st, just like everyone who matched in the first iteration.

You can choose not to apply during the second iteration of the match and instead take a year to improve your application. You could spend this year doing research, get a master's degree, or take clinical electives to improve your application. In this case you would be eligible to re-apply in the first iteration of the match in the following year. If you're only interested in one area of medicine, then this might be the right answer for you. I'd recommend calling the programs that you were interested in originally and asking why you didn't match.

MCCQE I

This is a day-long computer-based exam in two parts. The first is a series of multiple-choice questions from all areas of medicine. The computer adapts to your ability, so that after every twenty questions, your level of ability is calculated and you're given twenty more questions, chosen by the computer's algorithm to match your skill level. If you do better, the questions get harder. If you start answering them wrong, the questions get easier. For this reason, many people leave the exam not really knowing how they've done. The second half of the exam consists of mini-clinical scenarios, and it's your task to give a differential diagnosis, order tests, or interpret findings. Overall, it's an exhausting and expensive day.

Due to the exhausting and expensive nature of the day, make sure you've prepared adequately so you never have to do it again.

There's a famous publication fondly known as *The Toronto Notes* that has summarized vast amounts of knowledge for the MCCQE I. When you're studying, remember that each section of medicine (e.g., Surgery, paediatrics, internal) is worth just as much as every other section. There's also a section on statistics, public health, and ethics. You can get some easy marks by memorizing how to calculate sensitivity, specificity, and the positive predictive value.

When I prepared for this test, I went through a series of questions from the *Pre-Test* series, so I would be well-versed on answering multiple-choice questions. This series of books also spends a great deal of time explaining why the other choices are not correct, which makes it a very useful book indeed. In general, this is not a test that you can cram for. There really is just too much information. Take your time, study throughout clerkship, brush up on the charts and statistics you need, and then go do it. You'll come home exhausted so go out and eat with your fellow classmates. You all need a break.

The Beautiful Six Weeks

After you graduate from medical school, there are six beautiful weeks of freedom before residency. For me, it was the first real vacation time I'd had in three years. You are in the precocious *lala* land of being a qualified doctor but being unable to work as one. It's a great time to travel for most people. Me, I went to Costa Rica, rented a 4x4, and drove across the country speaking the little Spanish I knew. I caught up on much needed sleep. I didn't have a pager to go off. I didn't even have an alarm clock. It was probably one of the best trips of my life.

When you're planning your beautiful six weeks, remember that you need to be back in the country a few days before residency actually starts, which is July 1st across the country. There are usually some mandatory orientation days prior to the start.

(I once heard someone saying to never go to the hospital on July 1st because the place is filled with new doctors…July 2nd is obviously much safer!)

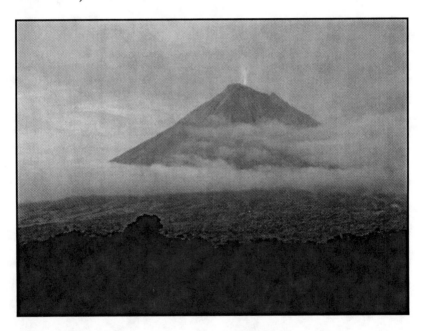

Hiking in Costa Rica during my beautiful six weeks

PART IV: BLOOD, SWEAT AND TEARS— RESIDENCY

Is there a doctor in the house?

CHAPTER 13: THE NEW RESIDENT

The Transition to PGY1

YOU'VE made it. You've graduated from medical school. You and your friends will call each other "Dr. So-and So" while you try out your new title. You have "Dr." before your name on your credit card, but you may appear too young to use it. Your family and friends are proud of you. You've gone out celebrating with your classmates and are ready to bravely face the new world of responsibility and decision-making that go along with your M.D.

I'll be honest. Starting PGY1 is extremely intimidating. You'll be expected to be on call on your own. You'll be covering patients you've not yet met. You'll be expected to manage acute situations, explain choices to patients and families, and teach clerks.

The first time I was on call from home, I wanted to drive in for every call I got, afraid to manage simple conditions over the phone without seeing the patient first. However, I quickly learned what I was comfortable with, and what I was not.

The first time I was on call in-house, I was covering surgery. There were only three doctors in the hospital – me, covering all surgical patients, and a resident each covering medicine patients and the intensive care unit. I had two cases of post-operative delirium, one that required security to be called because the patient was attacking the nurses with his IV pole. It's daunting to get a phone call saying there's a violent patient on the floor, "and you better get down here and do something about it!"

But I adjusted, learned to manage situations that had once scared me, and became comfortable with my role. And you will too. I have a vivid memory of being a clerk doing my medicine rotation, and watching my senior manage a woman with acute shortness of breath. She was frightened and the nurses and her family were worried about her, but my senior was able to take charge and manage the situation. I remember saying to him, "How does that happen? When do you start to know what to do when it's right there in your face?" He told me it comes with time. As I completed my first year of residency, I was on call for medicine and managing a woman who was very short of breath. She had lung cancer, COPD, and a probable pulmonary embolism. While I was organizing her care, the clerk I was with said to me, "Are you PGY1? I can't imagine being able to do this in a year. How does it happen?" I realised that I'd come full-circle. It does happen. You'll grow and become the doctor you want to be. Some things will always scare you and there will always be more to learn. But you'll become experienced, the clinical picture will become clearer, you'll be able to take care of people in an emergency, and suddenly you'll be doing things that used to terrify you.

I grew a lot during my first year as a doctor. Most people I talk to say that they feel much more comfortable with acuity in general after PGY1. Some hints for PGY1 survival:

1. Know who's backing you up. You should never be in the position of having no senior doctors to call on. Usually this is a senior resident but it may be a staff person. Find out who they are, and how to contact them.

2. Some seniors or staff might say things to you like, "Don't call me unless it's important" which might make you second guess if you should call them to ask a question. If you're worried about a patient, or ever feel like you're in over your head, it's the ethical choice to call the senior for back up. It's reasonable for them to assume that you've worked the patient up to the extent of your abilities and started some sort of initial management. And it's reasonable for you to assume that they'll provide recommendations.

3. Use your resources. This includes both material and personal. If you have a question and the time available, look it up. This not only provides a great learning experience (reading around the

patient), but also allows you to provide better care for your patient. If you read something that seems unfamiliar, talk to your senior before initiating treatment. Know where you can turn for help. If you're wondering how to convert one type of oral steroid to another type of IV steroid, call the pharmacy. If you don't know how to adjust the amino acids in someone getting TPN (total perenteral nutrition), call the dietician. If you're concerned that someone is being abused but don't know how to proceed, call a social worker. If you're called by a nurse and don't know what to do, don't be afraid to ask the nurses what medication people usually use, or what tests are usually ordered. They also usually know what type of management a particular staff person prefers, (e.g., one type of pain medication or antihypertensive over another) and will guide you in the right direction. Make the nurses your allies! Nurses really do not like "doctoritis." Whatever you do, don't give off the impression that you think you're better than they are. These are the people who have the power to page you over and over again in the middle of the night! It's respectful and more enjoyable to try to develop good working relationships with all of the other healthcare workers on a team. These professionals are experts in their respective fields and are extremely helpful in complex cases. Being able to identify issues and find people who can help solve them is part of the role of manager that doctors take on.

4. I found the paperwork the worst part of PGY1. As the most junior doctor on the team you'll be delegated all of the paperwork that requires a doctor's signature. Sometimes you'll need to call the radiologist on call if you want to do a CT, and sometimes you'll just fill out the form and leave it on the ward clerk's desk to fax it down. As frustrating as it is at first, it's not so bad once you figure out the system. Go get a coffee and find a time to do it all in one go if possible, and fill out things pre-emptively when you can. For example, discharge summary forms start with the patient's past medical history and reason for admission, which you can fill out when they're admitted, even if you don't have a diagnosis yet. Don't let your dictations build up; do them when people are sent home, otherwise you'll have to run around looking for the chart in medical records. Sometimes it's helpful to carry with you a bunch of common request forms, such as diagnostic imaging, EKG, and consult forms. This way, if a

patient needs a chest X-ray that morning, you can just pull it out and fill out the form when you need it.

5. Take the opportunity to teach. You were a clerk not so long ago, so do for your clerks what you liked your good residents to do for you. It keeps things interesting, consolidates your own learning, and contributes to a positive team atmosphere.

6. Don't say anything you wouldn't want people to hear. Being a resident really is quite stressful, and it's normal to want to have gripe sessions to get things off your chest about patients or other staff at the hospital. Do this somewhere private with people you trust. Be especially careful not to say anything negative in public about other doctors, nurses or patients. If you disagree with another professional's opinion and are asked about it, instead of saying, "Well, they don't know what they're talking about," state your opinion without degrading the esteem of the other professional. First of all, you were not there when the initial observation was made, so you don't really know the whole story from that perspective. Second, it breaks down the team concept and makes everyone look bad. Degrading that trust can impede communication, which can ultimately affect patient care.

7. Get help if you need it. Residency is mentally, physically, and emotionally exhausting. It's already been stated in this book that doctors experience higher than average levels of depression, anxiety, substance abuse, and suicide. If you're overwhelmed, talk to your program director about it. You'll not be the first resident who took some time off if you decide you need it, nor will you be the last. Many resident programs have services available for residents and doctors who are experiencing extreme stress.

8. Get a family doctor. It's amazing how many residents are surrounded by friends who are doctors but do not have a family doctor. Your family doctor can provide an unbiased opinion of your health and well-being, as well as a sense of confidentiality, which your friends cannot. It's especially important to have a family doctor if you're experiencing high levels of stress, are thinking of becoming pregnant, or have a medical condition that requires follow-up.

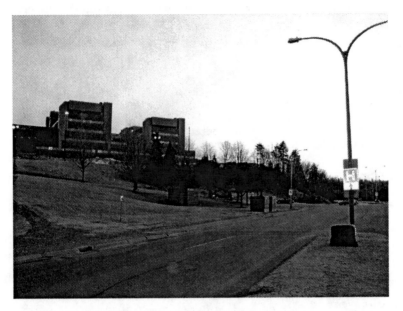

Sunrise over the Saint John Regional Hospital on my way to work. One of the perks of being a doctor is the unusual number of sunrises you'll see!

Doc Talk

The first day as an R1 was hard for me because I'd taken a year off to do my masters. I sat down and told the staff person that I hadn't been on call in a while. He chuckled and told me not to worry. It was there that I decided I'm here, I have to be competent. I realised that I can push myself, I can do more. If I'm stuck in one realm I can move to another. I realised I knew how to handle patients.

–Dr. Rickesh Sood, 2nd year family medicine resident

I have a family member who's a doctor and she absolutely hated residency. So she insisted that before I apply for residency I read "House of God." But it's the most misogynistic and awful book. The first few months of residency were hard for me because I didn't love it. Residency is a rollercoaster of highs "I intubated that twenty-eight week-er" and lows "Oh no, I bolused the wrong fluid and the surgery is now delayed."

–Dr. Jennifer Graham, 1ˢᵗ year paediatrics resident

The Happy Robot

Being on call is exhausting. There are times when it feels like your pager will never stop going off. There are consults in emergency, phone orders, and acute patient situations. After working all day, putting in another nineteen hours until you can go home can wear you down, especially when you know you won't be going home until noon the next day. It's easy to develop a negative attitude when you're tired, stressed, and surrounded by people who are in pain or dangerously sick.

As a clerk, I remember following around my internal medicine senior resident one particularly busy night, and there was a serious crisis, page after page. He was able to keep his cool, had a wonderful attitude, and never became bitter or upset. I asked him how he managed this, and he told that during his first year in residency he hated being on call, complained a lot about it, and was generally miserable. He then realized that doing heavy call was a fact of life while he trained in internal medicine before doing what he really wanted to do - a fellowship in rheumatology. So he decided to keep a positive attitude throughout his residency. He said that when he was really tired, he just decided he had to be the "Happy Robot" and make an effort to complete each task as positively as possible. This decision to maintain a cheerful disposition made his call much more bearable.

When I was on rotations as a first-year resident and had a particularly stressful call, I would try to be that Happy Robot; someone who was cheerful, respectful, energetic, and could go-go-go. This purposeful attitude decision made the call easier for me, and helped me provide better care to my patents.

Communication While on Call

"There is only one cardinal rule: one must always listen to the patient."
—Dr. Oliver Sacks

People who are sick in hospitals are often afraid and angry, and it's not uncommon for them to lash out at you, as the clerk or junior resident attending to them. Again, this can be difficult when you yourself have had little sleep, don't know the patient or the family because you're covering overnight, and have a number of critical scenarios happening concurrently. In this situation, it's important to remember that you, the family members, and the patient are all on the same side. You want them to get better, have less pain, and be healthier. Keep reminding yourself of that, and express it to the people who are angry. Although they may be quite upset, remember it's usually from the stressful situation they're in—not you. Try to put yourself in their position and imagine what the patient or their family is worried about. Imagine how they feel. When a patient or family member speaks harshly to you, try to remember that they probably would have spoken that way to anyone in your similar position, and that it's not intended for you personally. If people are directly insulting, it's okay to state that you do not appreciate being spoken to in that manner. If someone is aggressive or threatening, remove yourself from the situation, and if necessary, call security. You should never feel in danger. I once had a patient lunge at me and try to hit me. He was stable, so I refused to see him until he'd settled down and I knew security was nearby.

This is an example of how I worked with a family that was very upset while I covered internal medicine. It was a very busy night and I was taking care of a very sick woman who was having acute shortness of breath. It was ten at night and I was paged by a nurse saying that the family of another patient was there. They had some concerns and they wanted to speak with a doctor. They had expected a specific diagnostic test to be done that day and it hadn't been done, and the family, understandably, wanted to know why. I did not know the family or the patient. I did not know why the test was ordered in the first place or why it had been cancelled. But I was the one who was called to speak to the family, because I (a lowly PGY1) was the only doctor available. I walked into the room, introduced myself, and told them that I understood they had some questions for me. I let them know that I'd been unable to come right away because I'd had a patient who was quite sick, and that I had come as soon as possible.

A daughter and son-in-law of the patient were standing at the patient's bedside. They looked worried, tired, angry, and frustrated. We went to a private room to talk, and they told me that a test had been cancelled and they wanted to know why. The patient's daughter stated that if the test was not going to be done that she wanted to take her dad home so he could die peacefully there instead of having him lie around the hospital, waiting for some test. I told her that I understood her frustration. I let her know that I was aware of her concern for her father's comfort. I sympathized with her regarding the unexplained cancellation of the test her father was supposed to have been given. Both she and her husband expressed their anger and frustration, and I continued to empathize with her.

I let her know that I didn't know what was happening with the test because I had not met her father before. After speaking with the ward clerk, it became apparent that the test had been booked for a different date, but for some reason the family had been told it was going to happen today. I went back, told the family what had happened, and continued to express my sympathy. I told the woman that I would leave a note with the morning ward clerk to call about finding out if another test had been booked. I told them I would speak directly with her father's doctor in the morning about what had happened so he could be available to them to answer specific questions. I also asked them if there was anything else I could do for them, or any questions I could answer. By the end of the conversation, the family members were thanking me for what I had done and apologizing for speaking so angrily to me.

In the end, I didn't do anything medically for this family. But a major part of being a doctor is caring for people's emotional and social well-being. This conversation could have been disastrous - I knew nothing about what was going on, the family was frustrated, the father was extremely sick and possibly near death, and everyone was tired. There was also no way to actually solve the problem at ten at night. But I respected and empathized with the feelings and fears of the family, reassured them that they had not been forgotten, and was honest about how much I knew about the situation and what I could do for them at that moment. I gave them a chance to provide ideas about what they thought was going on. I did not accept any blame for what was happening (as there was nothing I had done to cause the situation), nor did I blame anyone else. Instead, I deflected the anger towards the situation itself. I made a plan, meagre as it was, followed through on it, and communicated with the family. When patients and families are angry, try to visualize yourself sitting on the same side of the table with them. Look at a problem together. This is especially important when you yourself have been up all night, are stressed, and have multiple issues on your mind such as other critical patients.

There's a lot of truth in the theory that when under stress, people cannot always take in detailed information. While communicating, you may need to reiterate basic facts, break things down to the bottom line, and try not to become too technical. Retention while stressed can be low, so, if necessary, ask the patient to repeat back what they understand is going on. It's okay to say that you don't know when you don't know.

If you're to blame for the situation, take responsibility for it, speak directly to the patient and the family, do what you can to rectify it, and tell someone senior about it. Not only is this your legal and ethical responsibility, but you probably will not make the same mistake again and will sleep much better at night.

The Rest of Your Life: Marriage, Children, Travel

The road of medicine can sometimes seem like some sort of all-consuming path. You were a person before you became a doctor; you wanted to fall in love, maybe have some kids, and see the world. People who go into medicine tend to have big dreams and big plans, and then all of a sudden your life is so completely consumed by medicine that it makes it hard to remember what else you wanted to do with your life. I want to assure you that life, kids and the rest of it are compatible with becoming a doctor. Many people were engaged or married during medical school while I was a medical student (I was married three months before starting medical school) and many more have done the same since starting residency. You should certainly not overlook the problems associated with being married to a medical student or doctor (I myself have just returned from three months in New Brunswick, while my husband continued school in Halifax – I drove home to see him every other weekend), but many people do it successfully.

As for children, some people are already parents when they begin medical school, but the most popular and logistically plausible time to have kids is during residency. Residents tend to be people in their twenties and thirties, which is a pretty normal time to want to start a family. Residency programs in Canada all have maternity leave with almost full pay for three months. Some programs will allow you to take three months for maternity leave without requiring you to make it up, and you can still finish your program the year you planned to. Some people choose to take six months or even a year. It really is an ideal time to take leave since your position will not be jeopardized. There is debate over what residency year is the ideal time for pregnancy, but most would say some time after second year, because the brunt of heavy call is over. However, people have had lovely, fantastic kids born in all years of residency!

Travel can be incorporated into your residency program. You can attend international conferences and attach vacation days to the end of it, giving you two weeks in another country. Most programs have some sort of elective time, and it's possible to spend some of this time working and traveling overseas. Practicing medicine in a developing country could remind you why you decided to go to medical school in the first place. Most programs also have research time available, which you could spend traveling and working on a study or survey. Of course, if you need more time to just travel without the work responsibilities, you generally get four weeks a year for vacation. If you plan things in advance, you may be able to group a large amount of this time together, allowing you to spend twenty days backpacking through Thailand.

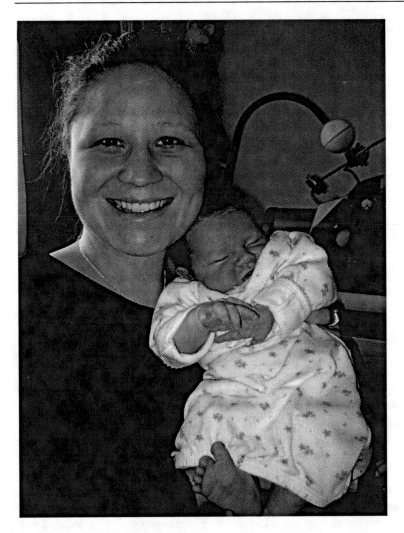

Dr. Sandra DeMontbrun, 3rd year general surgery resident, and her baby girl Devon.

Am I Stuck in This Field of Medicine?

To answer your question simply, the answer is no. The match can seem extremely final; there is a legally-binding contract, and the match algorithm makes everyone else's position depends on yours. If you think you're in the wrong field of medicine and want to switch, try to do it as early as possible in your training. Your ability to change programs depends largely on funding. When you receive a residency position, you get a certain number of years of funding provided to you depending on the program and location. Speak to the residency director of the program you're interested in. It's much easier to switch residency programs within a university than between universities. This means that if you're currently at Queen's in anaesthesia and want to switch to general surgery at Queen's, this is easier than switching to anaesthesia at Western. Intra-provincial switches are also easier than inter-provincial switches, meaning that it's far easier to change to another school in the same province than it is to change to a school farther away. Changing to a program of equal or shorter length is far easier than switching to one of greater length. All switches are easier if the money is already available to the university.

Some of the rotations you've already completed up to that point in your current residency can be counted towards your new residency. For this reason, if you're going to switch, do it early to save you time. However, I've heard anecdotally of people switching to family medicine as late as four or five years into a specialty!

I've heard from an unofficial source that the University of Toronto makes switching from one five-year program to another fairly easy if made during the first year of residency. This doesn't apply to all five-year programs, but apparently radiology, general surgery, ob-gyn, and paediatrics are relatively easy to switch between.

If you find you don't like your field of medicine, there are other options. Family medicine is the most flexible from this position. There are a multitude of family medicine fellowships that can dramatically change the way you practice medicine. For example, I've met family doctors who specialize in geriatrics and spend most of their time doing good old-fashioned house calls. Some people also find a renewed sense of interest in their career by choosing to work exclusively internationally. Others pursue a masters or PhD and divide their time evenly between working on basic science research and seeing patients. The possibilities within medicine really are quite broad if you think creatively about it, but for some people there's still a chance that this really isn't what you want to do anymore.

Some people get halfway through residency and discover that they hate medicine. They're overworked, overtired, and want out.

They feel trapped financially because they're in debt up to their eyeballs and the only way to pay it off in a timely fashion is to gain employment as a physician. Sometimes they choose to work for a few years doing locums (filling in for other physicians who are away) until their debt is paid off, and then go out and do something else with their life.

The MCCQE Part II

Yes, here it comes again, another very expensive exam (about $1,500) that you are required to take and pass. Most people do it during their second year of residency, although you can technically take it any time before you finish your residency. The application for the exam is due in the spring, and there's a very expensive penalty if you do not register in time. For the most part, it's up to you to find out about the deadlines and submit your application. Your residency program may not send out reminders about this.

The exam itself is an OSCE that takes place sometime in October. You'll be given a date and time, either a Saturday or Sunday. The exam for each day is the same across Canada, and so you may be sequestered for up to three hours afterwards to protect the academic integrity of the exam. During this time you will not have access to phones or computers.

The exam covers all areas of medicine from surgery to paediatrics and is done in two parts. The first is a set of ten-minute stations in which you have both a patient and an examiner. There will be a short scenario written and posted on the door, such as: "David M. is a twenty-four-year-old man who was found stabbed outside a bar. Manage." You'll walk into the room and there'll be an actor with fake blood and wounds, unconscious, or in pain. You might have a nurse available to give orders to. You generally have to stabilize the patient, figure out what needs to be addressed, order the correct lab work, and consult the right departments. You might also have a scenario where there's a patient who wants to quit smoking or is worried about their child. In many of the ten-minute stations, you'll be told some new information or be asked a question by your examiner after nine minutes. Often it's of an ethical nature: you're treating an alcoholic and the nurse tells you that his girlfriend is on the phone and wants to know how he's doing. The patient does not want his girlfriend to know what's happening to him. What do you tell the nurse?

The second part of the exam is a set of five-minute clinical scenarios, followed by five minutes in which to answer questions, interpret or order lab results, and to potentially write out a differential diagnosis. The scenarios are as varied as they are for the ten-minute stations, but often you only do a history or a physical exam, and not both.

The pass-rate for this exam is 95%, and you're scored on both your ability to manage the scenario medically and your rapport and appropriateness with the patient.

I studied for this exam with a group of friends and we quizzed each other and practiced running mock codes on each other. The questions from year to year tend to be recycled, and there are lots of circulating "packages" that have copies of exam questions dating back to the mid 1990's. The frustrating thing about this exam is that unless you're in family medicine, you've probably been away from a number of these topics for a long period of time. For example, because of the specialty I went into, I hadn't examined a shoulder in two years. However, musculoskeletal injuries were fair game for this exam, so I had to review the examination of different joints. It's hard to juggle the studying you're supposed to be doing for your own residency program along with having to review all of internship and medical school. I'd recommend doing it as soon as you can (in your second year). Prepare for it and do it well. Get it over with and then focus on your residency.

CHAPTER 14: YOU, THE PHYSICIAN

Staying Human

AS I write this I'm post-post call, the day after recovery from staying up all night; it's often the hardest day of the call schedule. I'm physically and emotionally exhausted from my Thursday night call. There were crisis after crisis, including a crash C-section to get out a transverse second twin with a dropping and then disappearing heart rate at four in the morning. Benodine was splashed on the mother's belly, we made a Pfannenstiel incision, and tore through each layer with a strength I didn't know I had. Fat. Facia. Rectus. Peritoneum. Ah, the uterus, no time to dissect off the bladder, slice, slice, my feet start to feel wet as my shoes were soaked through to the socks with blood. We pulled out what looked like a dead baby. I scooped her up and ran to the awaiting paediatric team, and as I did so I saw the child flutter her little eyes. We closed each layer carefully, and the patient was awakened and started on high-dose antibiotics. Crisis averted. The mother is alive. The baby is alive. I walk out of the OR and the husband and now father is standing in the hallway. He can see into the OR with the bloody sheets piled on the floor. He sees me standing there soaked in his wife's blood up to my knees. I tell him that his wife's going to be all right. He says to me, "There sure is a lot of blood," and just stands there. I gently guide him into the recovery room to be with his wife. I then go change my pants and socks, and walk into the next room where there's another patient I need to care for.

How do we handle this level of intensity? I often ask myself how I manage to take the terror and put it aside when there's a job that needs to be done. I ask myself how I manage not to laugh, cry, or scream when I realize what I've been a part of. Since starting residency I've had my share of dramatic moments. I once rode a gurney into the operating room, holding a baby's head off his cord during a prolapse. This is when the umbilical cord is being crushed by the baby's head, effectively cutting off his circulation. As I rode that gurney with the baby's head in my hand, I knew that it could become disabled or die if I let go before a C-section could be performed. I had a patient who stood up after a twenty minute conversation and died standing there, in front of me, of a massive pulmonary embolism. I've reached down a broken throat with a crumbling jaw to clear an air way. I've put pads on a patient's chest and zapped him with electricity to reset his heart, only to have him sit straight up and scream, later remembering nothing. I've held the heads of trauma victims to keep their spine straight as they are rolled to examine their back. I've stood in the operating room, squeezing the open uterus of a woman with a bleeding disorder as we call down to the lab over and over to bring platelets and blood, knowing that until it arrives, literally holding her together is the only option available to keep her from bleeding out. And there was that horrible night in the emergency room, when I diagnosed two people with cancer.

There are other days when there is no drama: just clinics, paperwork, some people glad to see you, others not so glad. You do a good job, make it through your day, feel good about it, and come home again.

There are days when there's nothing you can do to help. There are days when your patients are unhappy with you, when there's been a miscommunication somewhere along the line that makes everyone frustrated and grumpy, when you're torn between multiple responsibilities as your pager keeps going off for more to do.

You cannot be in more than one place at the same time. You only have two hands. It takes time to learn things. How do you keep it all together? How do you continue to be yourself?

For every low there really is a high. Those moments of terror are often reflected on as moments of real growth. That fear is translated into relief. The baby was okay. The bleeding stopped. You did the right thing. And here is where one of the true pleasures in medicine lies. The knowledge that you did it right, you did your best, and there's someone out there who's living a healthier life because you used your brain to change things for the better.

That being said, medicine does change you. I know that I've personally become more assertive and much less worried about confrontation. I have a greater sense of worry about the people I treat. I know that as my training goes on the outcome becomes more and more my personal responsibility. Sometimes I worry so much I cannot sleep. People use the expression "wanting to stay human" when they're referring to the constant sense of being overwhelmed, a sense that they're not themselves. And perhaps they use it too when they're disheartened by the workload. For some, perhaps they're so overworked and overtired that a certain numbness has set in. Most of the complaints I have myself, as well as those I hear from my colleagues, have much more to do with the politics of medicine than the doctoring itself. It's the conflicts between departments or the vicious comments you overhear. It's the forms to fill and the grumpy voice of another overworked person.

If you're constantly feeling inhuman, please get help. It doesn't have to be like this. Talk to your family doctor if you're depressed. Take time off if you need to. Re-evaluate your life and switch programs if you need to. You've worked so hard to get here. This is the dream you've chased for years.

Take care of yourself. Seek out people you can trust and talk to, stay close with old friends, and meet people outside of medicine. Use your vacation time, get a hobby, and try to talk about things other than medicine when you're together with your colleagues.

On days when I'm feeling overwhelmed, I've discovered that there's something very therapeutic about being good to someone else - it can sooth your own soul. You'll dislike who you've become the moment you start taking out your frustrations on your patients and colleagues. We're doctors. It's in our nature to reach out to someone, to make an action plan, to be helpful, to ease suffering. So do that with all your might.

To be honest, I never really liked the phrase "staying human" when discussing whatever it is that becoming a doctor does to you. I find the whole experience so *very human,* so very real, and so very true. This is how it really is. The people I meet are a cross-section of society and represent every walk of life. The experiences they're having are core experiences of their lives; they'll always remember being sick, being afraid, having hope, the birth of their child, the day they found out that their illness was treatable, or the day they found out that it wasn't. I've been honoured by patients feeling they can confide in me, cry in front of me, accept a hug from me, or share their joy and terrors with me. Becoming a physician teaches you how to read people. You will understand not only the way that someone moves when they have a kidney stone, but also the expression on someone's face when they are afraid to ask a question. This is the other true joy of medicine. The fact that you are human and are able to perceive apprehension, relief, and fear leads to a connection that helps people make better choices for themselves. These profound moments of connection enhance your understanding of the human experience, and make your world bigger, brighter, and more baffling.

The Truth about Being a Doctor

"It's supposed to be a secret, but I'll tell you anyway.
We doctors do nothing.
We only help and encourage the doctor within."
—Albert Schweitzer

The truth about being a doctor is that the wonderful parts really are as wonderful as you'd hoped. You meet amazing people and really are in a position to help them. It's fun to try to figure out what's going on and how to solve a problem. Each day truly has the potential for purpose. You really will get to know what it feels like to change a life. You will, however, be stressed to your limits. You'll have devastating failures. You'll be inhumanely tired. You'll find yourself living as a doctor even when you're relaxing, worrying about patients at night, talking shop with your friends. Is there life beyond medicine? What did you do with yourself before you went to medical school?

Your pager will go off and you'll want to throw it across the room because you really need to sleep. You'll have to get up anyway. You'll have to prove yourself to every single team of people you work with. Your actions at work will always matter. The truth is, it's more of everything than I ever imagined it could be - the highs higher, the lows lower. Most people I speak to say that the truth about this profession is hard to express, hard to pass on. Despite the pressure and the workload, though, there's nothing else they'd rather do. It's truly an amazing ride.

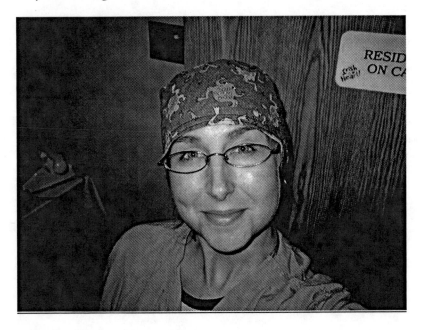

The author on call: greasy hair hidden conveniently under scrub cap

PART V: ENGLISH MEDICAL SCHOOLS—WEST TO EAST

CHAPTER 15: QUICK REFERENCE

H ERE'S a compilation of information on medical schools, east to west, at the time of publication. All information was obtained directly from official medical school websites, as well as OMSAS, the official central application site for Ontario medical schools. This took an unbelievably long time to compile, so hopefully I will have saved you some time. If information on a certain school is missing, it's because I could not find it from an official source.

Remember that requirements change from year to year, and they can even change within the same application cycle. I hope that this section gives you an idea of what medical schools are looking for, what type of GPAs and MCAT scores to strive for, and what the competition is like. I still urge you to confirm any pertinent information with the official websites of the schools, because I cannot guarantee accuracy. This is only an overview, a place to start. If you're seriously considering applying to a school it's a good idea to read as much as you can about it, or even call them directly, to better understand their admission criteria and teaching philosophy.

There is also a publication online here:

http://www.afmc.ca/docs/2005AdBk.pdf

This publication provides additional statistics in regards to medical school applications. Not all information on this website will be up-to-date. At the time of publication, the document was from 2005.

Quick List:
Schools that have no required courses:

Calgary
Western
McMaster
Northern Ontario
Dalhousie

Schools that do not require the MCAT:

Ottawa
Northern Ontario School of Medicine
McMaster (*requires the verbal reasoning section of the MCAT only*)

Schools that are 3 years in length:

Calgary
McMaster

Schools with some aspect of problem-based learning

Dalhousie
Ottawa
McMaster
Toronto
Queen's
Western
Northern Ontario
University of Alberta

Schools that interview using the Multiple Mini Interview:

Saskatchewan
Calgary
Manitoba (possibly)
McMaster
Northern Ontario

CHAPTER 16: INDIVIDUAL SCHOOL REQUIREMENTS

University of British Columbia Faculty of Medicine

Information source: http://www.med.ubc.ca

Location: Vancouver, BC.
Contact information: http://www.med.ubc.ca

Office of the Dean
317 - 2194 Health Sciences Mall
Faculty of Medicine
The University of British Columbia
Vancouver, BC V6T 1Z3

Telephone: 604-822-2421
Fax: 604-822-6061

Number of seats: 224 total. 176 seats are in the Vancouver Fraser Medical Program, 24 seats are in the Island Medical Program, and 24 seats are in Northern Medical Program.

What are my chances? 1 in 7. There are 1,580 applicants for 224 available seats. Residents of BC are preferred. Only a few out-of-province students are admitted each year.

Duration of degree: 4 years

Tuition: $14,280

How do I apply? Online through UBC medicine website:
http://www.med.ubc.ca/education.htm

Application deadline: The application is made available in early June
and is due in early September.

Admission Criteria

Number of credits: 90 by April 30th.

Required courses: Six credits each of English, biology, general
chemistry, organic chemistry, and biochemistry. Behavioural sciences
courses, statistics, and physics are recommended but not required.

Required GPA: 70% required to apply (or 2.8/4.0). The average
admission grade is 83%.

How they calculate your GPA: The average GPA is calculated by
averaging all university courses attempted, with the last sixty credits
and prerequisite courses weighing more heavily than the rest.

MCAT: Mean MCAT scores of the class entering 2005:
VR 9.35
PS 10.21
WS P
BS 10.66

http://www.med.ubc.ca/__shared/assets/2009_Class_Statistics1024.
pdf

Personal: A supplemental form is filled out if you're invited to
interview. Qualities including well-roundedness, motivation, maturity,
and concern for human welfare are valued.

Letters of recommendation: These are only requested at the time of
invitation to interview.

Interview style: Standard interview panel.

Curriculum description:

Year 1:
Priniciples of Human Biology
Host Defense and Infection
Cardiovascular
Pulmonary, Fluids and Electrolytes and Renal GU.
There are also three longitutial courses - Patient and Society, Family
Practice Continuum, and Clinical Skills.

Year 2: Musculoskeletal and Locomotor, Blood and Lymphatics,
Gastrointestinal, Endocrine and Metabolism, Integumentary (skin),
Brain and Behaviour, Reproduction, and Growth and Development.
During the second year you continue the longitutinal courses of
Patient and Society, Family Practice Continuum, and Clinical Skills at
a more advanced level.

Year 3: Students spend four to eight weeks in a rural or
underserviced area and start clerkship. Clerkship rotations include:

- general surgery
- emergency
- internal medicine
- paediatrics
- obstetrics and gynecology
- psychiatry
- orthopedic surgery
- opthomology
- dermatology
- anesthesiolgy

Students have an opportunity for elective time during this period.

Year 4: Students have selective (at UBC) and elective (anywhere) time from September to December. Year four also has a multidisiplinary component covering areas such as phamacology, the doctor-patient relationship, critical appraisal, and the legal and ethical aspects of medicine.

Special programs or opportunities: An M.D./PhD is availible.

Information for special applicants:

Graduate students: The same evaluation criteria are used for graduate students as for undergraduatae students. Your thesis must be completed by July 1st the summer prior to admission.

Aboriginal applicants: UBC encourages Aboriginal students to apply. You should contact the Aboriginal Programs Coordinator by email at james.andrew@ubc.ca or by telephone at (604) 822-3236.

If applying as an Aboriginal student, there's an extra application package which is considered by the Aboriginal Admissions Subcommittee.

Faculty of Medicine, University of Calgary

Information source: ucmedapp@ucalgary.ca

Location: Calgary, Alberta

Contact information:
Office of Admissions,
University of Calgary
Faculty of Medicine
3330 Hospital Drive NW
Calgary, Alberta
T2N 4N1
ucmedapp@ucalgary.ca

Number of seats: 125

What are my chances? 1 in 12.2. In the 2005/2006 cycle, there were 1,532 applicants for 125 positions. 85% of seats are reserved for residents of Alberta. Only 15% are for out-of-province students.

Duration of degree: 3 years

Tuition: $12,788

How do I apply? Online through the University of Calgary faculty of medicine website:

http://files.myweb.med.ucalgary.ca/files/62/files/unprotected/Applicants_Manual_for_On-Line_Application.pdf

Application deadline: November 1st

Admission Criteria

Number of credits: At least two years of full time university by the time you start medical school. It's preferred that you take 5 full courses (or 10 half courses), but 4 full courses (or 8 half courses) is acceptable.

Required courses: Calgary does not have any specific required courses but does strongly recommend the following courses:

2 semesters each of biology, chemistry, English, organic chemistry, biochemistry, and physiology
1 semester of psychology, sociology, or anthropology
1 semester of calculus or statistics

Required GPA: To apply, the required GPA for Albertans is 3.2, and for non-Albertans it's 3.6. Non-Albertans are invited to an interview based on an algorithm that takes into account a weighted GPA as well as the biological sciences and verbal reasoning section of the MCAT. Recently, the averaged weighted GPA for students invited to interview was 3.79.

How they calculate your GPA: The average of your best two years of full time university is used to calculate your weighted GPA. Summer courses are not counted.

MCAT: (from 2005 data)

VR:10.48
PS: 10.10
Writing sample: Q
BS: 11

Personal: The following are considered in your application:

employment history
extracurricular activities
sports
hobbies
travel
leadership
arts
volunteerism
awards
application essay

Letters of recommendation: Three letters of recommendation are required.

Invitation for interview: Applicants are invited to interview based on the following criteria:

entire academic record 50%
employment history and extracurricular activities 25%
MCAT 15%
personal essay 5%
reference letters 5%

Aboriginal applicants who meet the GPA cut-off of 3.2 for Albertans and 3.6 for non-Albertans will be invited to interview.
For Non-Albertans to be considered who are not of Aboriginal ancestry, the following algorithm is used to rank the applicants:

$$62.517 \,(GPA) + 12.122 \,(MCAT \; VR \; score) + 6.757 (MCAT \; BS \; score)$$

The top 125 students according to this algorithm are further reviewed by the admissions committee, meaning their application is then reviewed according to the above breakdown including GPA, MCAT, employment history and extracurricular activities, personal history, and reference letters. Recently, the lowest score to be reviewed was 449.13.

Interview style: Multiple Mini Interview plus an on-site essay

Curriculum description:

Year 1:

- integrated fever/sore throat, blood and gastrointestinal
- integrated musculoskeletal and special senses
- integrated cardiovascular and respiratory
- integrated renal-electrolyte and endocrine-metabolic

There are also longitudinal courses covering medical skills and research methods and evidence-based medicine, plus elective time in the first year of school.

Year 2:

- integrated neurosciences and aging
- integrated reproductive medicine and infant/child
- integrated mind and family

Second year also has a longitudinal medical skills course, as well as a longitudinal applied evidence-based medicine course. There's elective time and an introduction to clerkship.

Year 3:

Clerkship starts in April of your second year of medical school. Clerkship rotations include:

- general surgery
- internal medicine
- paediatrics
- obstetrics and gynaecology
- family medicine
- psychiatry
- anaesthesia
- elective time

Special programs or opportunities: Joint M.D./PhD as well as joint M.D./MA, M.D./MBA and M.D. MSc.

Information for special applicants:

Graduate students: Your graduate studies will be considered as part of your application as long it was full time, you took at least half a course, and you received a grade.

Aboriginal applicants: The same GPA cut-off criterion is used for general as well as Aboriginal applicants. However, all Aboriginal applicants who meet the cut-off will be interviewed.

University of Alberta

Information source: http://www.med.ualberta.ca

Location: Edmonton, Alberta.

Contact information:
2-45 Medical Sciences Bldg
114 Street & 87 Avenue
Edmonton, Alberta, Canada
T6G 2H7
Phone: (780) 492-6350
Fax: (780) 492-9531

Number of seats: 134
What are my chances? 1 in 8.2 This medical school usually receives about 1,100 applications. There are 134 seats. Students who are residents of Alberta have an advantage in that 85% of seats are reserved for them. The other 15% of seats are for non-Albertans.

Duration of degree: 4 years

Tuition: $10,387

How do I apply? Apply online through the university of Alberta medicine website.

Application deadline: November 1st, initial application.
November 15th, secondary application.

Admission criteria: Number of credits: at least two full years of
university while enrolled in a degree program. This means a total of 10
full credits.

Required courses:
general chemistry, 1 year; IB chemistry will count as half of this
requirement if you received a 6 or 7.
organic chemistry, 1 year
biology, 1 year (includes microbiology, zoology, genetics, botany,
physiology, bacteriology, immunology and entomology; IB biology will
count as half of this requirement if you received a 6 or 7)
physics, 1 year (make sure that it's an approved physics course, not an
astronomy, astrology, or music and high fidelity course. Contact U of A
if you're not sure if a physics course will be accepted before you take it
to avoid wasting your time and being extremely disappointed.)
English, 1 year; either a full year of English literature, or half a year each
of English literature and English composition. IB English will count as
half of this requirement if you received a 6 or 7.
statistics, 1/2 year.
biochemistry, 1/2 year.

GPA: If applying with four years of undergraduate work the average
GPA for all courses is 3.7, the average of the prerequisite courses stated
above is 3.83.

If applying with two or three years of undergraduate work, the average
GPA for all courses is 3.8 and the average of the prerequisite courses is
3.9

How they calculate your GPA: Both the straight GPA and the GPA of
prerequisite courses are taken into consideration. If more than four years
of undergraduate work are taken, the year with the lowest GPA is not
included in the calculation.

MCAT: If applying with four years of undergraduate work the average
MCAT is 10.76 with a Q in the writing sample. If applying with two or
three years of undergraduate work the average MCAT is 11.64 with a Q
in the writing sample. No score in a single section should be less than 7.

Personal: The admission committee evaluates you based on employment record, awards or achievements, leadership roles, volunteer work, and diversity of experiences.

Letters of recommendation: Two letters of reference are required.

Invitation to interview: Invitation to interview is based on cumulative GPA (15/70 points), prerequisite course average (15/70 points), MCAT score (15/70 points), MCAT writing sample (5/70), and personal attributes (20/70).

Interview style: Interviewed by a panel of 3 people. These people are often a layperson, a scientist, and a clinician.

Acceptance: The interview is given a score out of 25, and the letters of reference a score out of 5. These scores are added to the pre-interview score to make a final score out of 100. Students are ranked by this new score and offers of acceptance are made accordingly.

Curriculum description:

Years 1 and 2:

endocrinology, gastroenterology, cardio-pulmonary-renal, musculoskeletal, obstetrics/gynaecology/urology, neurology/organs of sense, oncology, infection/inflammation

Clerkship:

- general surgery
- internal medicine
- obstetrics and gynaecology
- paediatrics
- rural family medicine psychiatry
- anesthesia

Special programs or opportunities: The University of Alberta offers an M.D./PHD program as well as an M.D. with Special Training In Research (STIR), which is a program including 24 weeks of supervised research.

Information for special applicants:

Graduate students: If you're a graduate student (either a masters or a PhD), your grades during your graduate studies will be considered as long as you took a full year course during each year. Your thesis must be defended by June 15th if you want your masters or PhD considered as part of your application. The application committee may want to contact your defence committee so they can look at your thesis evaluation.

If you have a masters, one point is added to your application. With a PhD, you get three extra points.

Aboriginal student policy: Please contact: Coordinator, Native HealthCare Careers Program, 2-45 Medical Sciences Building, University of Alberta, Edmonton, Alberta, T6G 2H7. Telephone: (780) 492-9526, E-mail: ugme@med.ualberta.ca

University of Saskatchewan College of Medicine

Information source: http://www.medicine.usask.ca/

Location: Saskatoon, Saskatchewan.

Contact information:
http://www.medicine.usask.ca/
B103 Health Sciences Building
107 Wiggins Road
Saskatoon, SK S7N 5E5
Canada
Tel 306-966-6135 fax 306-966-6164
med.admissions@usask.ca

Number of seats: 60
What are my chances? 6 seats are set aside for Aboriginal students. Up to 6 seats will be offered to out-of-province students.

Duration of degree: 4 years

Tuition: $11,460

How do I apply? Applications are available at:
http://www.usask.ca/medicine

Application deadline: December 1st.

Admission Criteria

Number of credits: At least two full years of university must be completed at the time of application. However, Saskatchewan students may apply during the second year, assuming they do well on final exams.

Required courses: Saskatchewan students must be enrolled in the Arts and Sciences Pre-Medical Program and have taken, biochemistry, biology, chemistry, organic chemistry, physics, English, and a full course in social sciences or humanities.

Required GPA: A minimum two-year average is 78% for residents of Saskatchewan. For out-of-province students the minimum average is 80%. The average grades of those accepted in 2005 was 89.19%.

How they calculate your GPA: The average of your two best years is used.

MCAT: To apply, a minimum of 8 or N is needed in each section. However, one grade of 7 or M is acceptable in any particular section. The average MCAT scores for the class starting in 2005 were:

BS:9.77
PS:9.73
VR 9.40
WS range M-S

Personal: Personal qualities are mainly assessed in the interview.
Letters of recommendation: Three letters of recommendation are required.
Invitation to interview: Unknown

Interview style: Multiple Mini Interview

Curriculum description:

Year 1:

- anatomy
- biochemistry and nutrition
- immunology
- physiology and neurosciences
- core pathology
- community service project or community experience

Year 2:

- systemic pathology
- microbiology
- genetics
- pharmacology
- clinical sciences in internal medicine and surgery

Year 3:

- community health and epidemiology
- obstetrics and gynaecology
- paediatrics
- psychiatry
- physical medicine and rehabilitation
- diagnostic imaging
- vertical themes of ethics and professionalism
- social accountability
- complimentary and alternative medicine opportunities such as SWITCH (student initiative toward community health) or international electives

Clerkship:

- anaesthesiology
- family medicine
- emergency medicine
- internal medicine
- surgery

- obstetrics and gynaecology paediatrics
- psychiatry

Special programs or opportunities: M.D./MSc and M.D./PhD

Information for special applicants:

Graduate students: If you're in a course-based program, your graduate grades will be added to your two best undergraduate years to calculate your average, or you can use just your two best undergraduate years, whichever is higher.

In a masters thesis-based program, your graduate grades will be added to your two best undergraduate years to calculate the average.
In a PhD, your graduate grades will count as one year and your best undergraduate year will count as a second year.

All degrees must be completed prior to starting medical school

Aboriginal students: 6 seats are reserved for Aboriginal Students - 3 of these are for Aboriginal students who are residents of Saskatchewan. Aboriginal students compete against each other, not the general application pool. There are opportunities for Aboriginal pre-med students through a medical mentorship program and scholarships.

University of Manitoba Faculty of Medicine

Information Source: http://umanitoba.ca/faculties/medicine/

Location: Winnipeg, Manitoba

Contact information:
Ms. Beth Jennings
Manager, Admissions & Student Affairs
Faculty of Medicine
260-727 McDermot Avenue
Winnipeg, MB R3E 3P5
Phone: (204) 789-3569
Fax: (204) 789-3929

Number of seats: 100

What are my chances? 1 in 8.2. There are 100 seats for approximately 815 applicants. 90% of the seats are for residents of Manitoba, and only 10% are for out of province students.

Duration of degree: 4 years

Tuition: $7,000

How do I apply? The application package is available on the website. It must be printed and mailed in.

Application deadline: October 2nd

Admission Criteria

Number of credits: You must be eligible to receive a bachelor's degree by June 30th of the year you want to apply.

Required courses: One full year of biochemistry and 18 credit hours of humanities or social sciences. There may be some exceptions to these 18 credit hours. Advanced placement with a minimum of 4 credits and international baccalaureate with a minimum of 5 credits are accepted.

Required GPA: An adjusted GPA of 3.6 or higher on a 4.5 point scale is required to apply.

How they calculate your GPA: GPA is on a 4.5 point scale. Graduate courses are not considered in calculating the GPA. An adjusted GPA is calculated by converting your percentage or letter grade to the 4.5 point scale. A certain number of courses will be dropped in calculating this average based on the number of credits you've completed, with more courses taken meaning you can drop more of your lowest grades in the calculation. The average adjusted GPA of those offered an interview in 2005 was 3.99.

MCAT: You cannot have scored lower than 7 in any section, or lower than an M on the writing sample. The average of your section scores (including your writing sample, where M=7 and T=14) must be at least 8 to apply. The average MCAT for those offered an interview in 2005 was 9.84.

Personal: Employment, extracurricular, volunteer, and community experiences are taken into consideration. A personal essay is required if you're invited to interview.

Letters of recommendation: Three letters of recommendation are required.

Invitation to interview: A combination of adjusted GPA and MCAT scores are used to choose who to invite to interview. Everyone who's a resident of Manitoba who meets the minimum screening requirements will be invited to interview. Students from out-of-province are ranked according to their adjusted GPA and MCAT, and about 60 of those with top scores will be invited to interview. In 2006, out-of-province students invited to interview had an average adjusted GPA of 3.95 and an MCAT of 10.75.

Interview style: Currently using a standard interview. However, they're considering switching to the Multiple Mini Interview.

Curriculum description: Mission statement: "The Mission of the Undergraduate Medical Education Program is to provide an environment which will assist students to become competent, caring, ethical physicians with the ability to think critically. This experience will prepare students to choose wisely their area of training, to successfully continue their education, and subsequently to meet responsibilities to their patients and society."
Year 1:

- Block I: Structure, Function, and Disease Mechanism, Population Health and Medicine.
- Block II: Human Development
- Block III: Cardiovascular, Ear Nose and Throat, Respiratory, Structure, Function, and Disease Mechanisms

Throughout this year there are longitudinal courses in:

- clinical skills
- problem solving
- medical humanities
- laboratory medicine
- stress management.

Year 2:

- Block IV: Endocrine and Metabolism, Kidney, Reproduction.
- Block V: Musculoskeletal, Ophthalmology, Neurosciences.
- Block VI: Blood and Lymph, Gastrointestinal, Dermatology

Throughout this year there are longitudinal courses in:

- clinical skills
- problem solving
- medical humanities
- laboratory medicine
- stress management.

Years 3 and 4:

Clerkship rotations include:

- general surgery
- internal medicine
- paediatrics
- obstetrics and gynaecology
- psychiatry
- family and community medicine
- emergency
- anaesthesia
- ear nose and throat
- ophthalmology
- dermatology
- community health sciences.

During the 4th year there's also ACLS, ATLS, and an LMCC review course as well as selective time and elective time.

Special programs or opportunities: B.Sc. Med (an undergraduate science degree earned during the summer months and concurrently with the regular M.D. program)

Information for special applicants:

Graduate students: The AGPA is calculated only using undergraduate marks. The graduate work will be considered an accomplishment to take into consideration along with your other extracurricular activities, letters of reference, personal essay, and interview.

Aboriginal students: Aboriginal students who are residents of Manitoba must have an adjusted GPA of at least 3.0. The MCAT score average must be at least 7, with no score less than 6 in any individual section. All applicants will be interviewed, and the selection criteria for admission are more heavily weighted towards the interview, letters of recommendation, extracurricular experiences, and personal essay.

Applicants who've worked in a health related field in direct contact with those receiving health or social welfare services for at least two years: These students are usually people who are nurses, social workers, physiotherapists, psychologists, or welfare workers. These special applicants have the same minimum criteria as the Aboriginal students stated above, and will all be invited to interview and have the same selection criteria more heavily weighted away from the adjusted GPA and MCAT.

Military: This category pertains to those whose positions are sponsored by the Department of National Defense. The criteria for application and selection criteria are the same as for Aboriginal students and those working in a health related field, as mentioned above.

The Schulich School of Medicine & Dentistry, University of Western Ontario

Information source: http://www.med.uwo.ca/, and http://www.ouac.on.ca/omsas/

Location: London, Ontario

Contact information:
Western, The Schulich School of Medicine & Dentistry
Admissions - Medicine

Kresge Building K1
519-661-3744
admissions.medicine@schulich.uwo.ca

Number of seats: 147

What are my chances? 1 in 17.2. There are 2,531 applications for the 147 available seats.

Duration of degree: 4 years

Tuition: $15,149

How do I apply? Apply through OMSAS online - http://www.ouac.on.ca/omsas/

Application deadline: Register by September 15th, submit by October 3rd.

Admission Criteria

Number of credits: You need to have completed a 4-year degree by the beginning of medical school.

Required courses: There are no required courses to apply to this medical school.

Required GPA: The minimum GPA needed to apply is 3.7.

How they calculate your GPA: Only years in which 5 full courses were taken during the academic term will be used to calculate your GPA average. Your best two years of undergraduate work will be used for this calculation (therefore you need at least two years where you went to school with a full course load). You must have the minimum GPA in each of the two undergraduate years that are being used to calculate your average.

MCAT:

For those applicants who attended high schools in Grey, Bruce, Huron, Perth, Oxford, Middlesex, Lambton, Chatham-Kent, Elgin, Norfolk, and Essex Counties, the minimum MCAT scores needed to be considered for interviews are as follows:

Biological Sciences - 8
Physical Sciences - 8
Verbal Reasoning - 8
BS, PS, VR combined total - 30
Writing sample - O

If you did not go to high school in any of these regions, the minimum MCAT score needed to be considered for an interview are as follows:

Biological Sciences - 10
Physical Sciences - 10
Verbal Reasoning - 10
BS, PS, VR combined total - 30
Writing Sample - Q

Personal: Ability to self-study, personal essay.

Letters of recommendation: Three letters are required.

Invitation to interview: The MCAT and GPAs are used to select students to attend an interview.

Interview style: Unknown

Curriculum description: Mission Statement: "The Schulich School of Medicine & Dentistry provides an outstanding education within a research intensive environment where tomorrow's physicians, dentists, and heath researchers learn to be socially responsible leaders in the advancement of human health."

Year 1: Introduction to Medicine, Infection and Immunity, Skin, Musculoskeletal System, Respiration and Airways, Heart and Circulation, Blood and Oncology, Patent-Centred Community methods, and Community Health I.

Year 2: Endocrine and Metabolism, Digestive System and Nutrition, Genitourinary System, Reproduction, Neurosciences, Eye and Ear, Psychiatry and Behavioural Sciences, Emergency Care, Community Health II, Patient-Centred Clinical Methods II.

Year 3: Clinical Clerkship:

- general surgery
- internal medicine
- paediatrics
- obstetrics and gynecology
- psychiatry
- family medicine

Year 4:

Elective and selective time, transition period courses.

Special programs or opportunities:

Combined M.D./PhD
Combined M.D./Engineering degree

Information for special applicants:

Graduate students: Grades achieved during a Masters or PhD will not be considered in calculating the GPA. Your graduate work has to be finished (with proof by a letter from your supervisor) prior to starting medical school.

Aboriginal students: There are 3 positions set aside for aboriginal students each year. Aboriginal students are evaluated on GPA, MCAT scores, and their involvement in the Aboriginal community.
Students from rural areas in south-western Ontario: Special consideration is given to students who are from south-western Ontario.

Michael G. DeGroote School of Medicine, McMaster University

Information source: http://www.fhs.mcmaster.ca/home.htm and http://www.ouac.on.ca/omsas/

Location: Hamilton, Ontario. 15 seats are in Kitchener-Waterloo

Contact information:
M.D. Admissions Office
McMaster University
Michael G. DeGroote School of Medicine
1200 Main Street West, M.D.CL - 3115
Hamilton, ON L8N 3Z5

Tel: (905) 525-9140 x22235
Fax: (905) 546-0349
Email: M.D.admit@mcmaster.ca

Number of seats: 162

What are my chances? 1 in 27.7. Competing for the 162 seats, there are more than 4,500 applicants each year. 80% of the interview positions are reserved for residents of Ontario, while only 10% are for out-of-province applicants.

Duration of degree: 3 years

Tuition: Unknown

How do I apply? Apply through OMSAS
http://www.ouac.on.ca/omsas/

Application deadline: Register by September 15th, submit by October 3rd.

Admission Criteria

Number of credits: By June 30th of the year you wish to start medical school, you need to have completed at least 3 years of undergraduate university.

Required courses: No courses are required.

Required GPA: Minimum GPA to apply is 3.00/4.00. The average GPA of those accepted is 3.88.

How to calculate your GPA: The simple average is taken of all courses ever taken. Each year is weighted equally. No years or courses (including summer courses) are dropped.
MCAT: The verbal reasoning section of the MCAT is required.

Personal: considered on your application are:

formal education
employment
volunteer activities extracurricular activities awards and accomplishments
autobiographical submission written responses to 5 questions

Letters of recommendation: Three letters of recommendation are required.

Invitation to interview: Invitation to interview is based on the average GPA and autobiographical submissions. (53% GPA, 43% autobiographical submission score, up to 4% can be added for graduate school experience).

Interview style: Multiple Mini Interview

Curriculum description:

Years 1 and 2: Medical foundations 1: Introduction to Determinants of Health and Oxygen Supply and Exchange (Cardio, Resp, Heme)
Medical Foundations 2: Homeostasis 1 (Energy Balance, GI, Endocrine, Nutrition)
Medical Foundations 3: Homeostasis 2: (Renal, Acid Base, Blood Pressure Control, Reproduction and Pregnancy, Genetics 1)
Medical Foundations 4: Host Defense, Neoplasia, Genetics 2
Medical Foundations 5: Movement Control, Interacting and Communicating (Behaviour, Nervous System, Musculoskeletal System)

Longitudinal concepts:

- pharmacology (metabolism of drugs)
- human development (early years and end of life)
- anatomy
- generalism
- pathology

Clerkship:

- family medicine,
- obstetrics and gynaecology
- psychiatry
- emergency
- paediatrics
- medicine
- anaesthesia
- surgery

Special programs or opportunities: In the future, McMaster may offer "streaming," wherein students can elect to participate in a variety of combined M.D. degrees, such as M.D./PhDs, or M.D./MBAs.

Information for special applicants:

Graduate students: Graduate work is not considered when calculating the mean GPA. However, those with a masters degree can add +0.01 to the scoring system used to choose who to invite to interview, and those with a PhD degree can add +0.04.

Students in a masters or PhD program must submit a letter from their supervisor saying that they're aware that the student is applying to medical school, and the degree needs to be completed by Oct 2nd, the application deadline.

Aboriginal students: Aboriginal students who would like to apply through the Aboriginal student application process need a letter of recommendation from a First Nation, band council, treaty, community, or organizational affiliation. People applying through this program need a minimum GPA of 3.00/4.00.

University of Toronto Medical School

Information source:
http://www.facmed.utoronto.ca/English/Undergraduate-Medical-Program.html and http://www.ouac.on.ca/omsas/
Location: Toronto, Ontario

Contact information:
Dr. Jay Rosenfield
Associate Dean, Undergraduate Medical Education
Faculty of Medicine, University of Toronto
Email: jay.rosenfield@utoronto.ca

Number of seats: 224

What are my chances? Less than 1 in 12.3. There are 2,764 applicants for 224 seats per last stats available.

Duration of degree: 4 years

Tuition: Unknown

How do I apply? Apply through OMSAS
http://www.ouac.on.ca/omsas/

Application deadline: Register by September 15th, submit by October 3rd.

Admission Criteria

Number of credits: Students are allowed to apply during or after the third year of university after completing 15 full credits.

Required courses: 2 full courses in the area of life sciences and 1 full course in humanities, social sciences, or languages.
The following courses are recommended but not required:

statistics, and 2 full courses that require expository writing.

Required GPA: Minimum GPA to apply is 3.6 on a 4.0 scale. The average GPA of those accepted is 3.87.

How they calculate your GPA: If you're applying during your third year of university, all your grades will be used equally to calculate your GPA. If you're applying after completing at least three years of university on a full-time basis, you can drop one course from your GPA calculation for each year of university. This means that if you're applying during your fourth year of university, you can have your lowest 3 full credits dropped from the calculation. Summer courses are not used in your

GPA calculation. If you did not attend university on a full-time basis you cannot drop any courses from the calculation.

MCAT: The MCAT is used as a flag only, and not as part of a calculation to decide who to invite to interview. Marks under 9 or under N may flag your application as unacceptable. The average MCAT marks of those accepted are as follows:

VR 10
PS 11
BS 11
WS Q

Personal: Formal education, employment, volunteer activities, awards, research, and "other." In the autobiographical sketch activities that demonstrate responsibility, altruism interest, creativity, commitment, and contribution to community as well as reliability, perseverance, and leadership are looked upon favourably. Applicants will also be evaluated on a personal essay.

Letters of recommendation: Three letters of recommendation are required.

Invitation to interview: The GPA (60%) and non-academic assessment (40%) is used to choose who to invite to interview.

Interview style: Traditional interview.

Curriculum description:

Year 1:

Structure and Function which includes:

* gross anatomy
* embryology
* histology
* cell biology
* biochemistry
* cardio-respiratory physiology haematology
* pharmacology and ethics nutrition and metabolism

- brain and behaviour

The longitudinal courses Art and Science of Clinical Medicine and Determinants of Community Health run concurrently.

Year 2:

Pathobiology of Disease
Foundations of Medical Practice, which includes:

- obstetrics and gynaecology
- paediatrics
- psychiatry
- family medicine
- general surgery
- medicine

The longitudinal courses Art and Science of Clinical Medicine and Determinants of Community Health are run concurrently.
Years 3 and 4:

Clerkship rotations include:

- medicine
- surgery
- obstetrics and gynaecology
- psychiatry
- family medicine (with ophthalmology and ENT)
- paediatrics
- emergency
- anaesthesia
- ambulatory medicine
- community health
- dermatology

Special programs or opportunities:
M.D./Ph.D

Information for special applicants:

Graduate students: Graduate students are considered separately from non-graduate students. The degree needs to be completed by June 29th the year you wish to enter medical school.

The minimum GPA needed to apply is 3.0 on a 4.0 scale. Graduate students are assessed on graduate course marks and publications as well as undergraduate marks, the MCAT, non-academic achievements, letters of reference, and the interview. Graduate students also need a letter from their supervisors evaluating their work and stating when the work will likely be finished.

Information source: http://meds.queensu.ca/school_of_medicine and http://www.ouac.on.ca/omsas/

Queen's School of Medicine

Information source: http://meds.queensu.ca/school_of_medicine and http://www.ouac.on.ca/omsas/
Location: Kingston, Ontario

Contact information:

Admissions Office: 613-533-330
Mailing Address:
Undergraduate Medical Education
68 Barrie Street, Queen's University
Kingston, Ontario, K7L 3N6
Fax: (613) 533-3190

Number of seats: 100

What are my chances? 1 in 22. There were 2,205 applicants for the 100 available seats.

Duration of degree: 4 years

Tuition: Unknown

How do I apply? Apply through OMSAS
http://www.ouac.on.ca/omsas/

Application deadline: Register by September 15th, submit by October 3rd.

Admission Criteria

Number of credits: Three years of study (fifteen full credits) in any university program.

Required courses: The equivalent of one full university credit in each of the following groups:

biological sciences, physical sciences, and humanities or social sciences

Required GPA: The most recent cut-off is an average GPA of 3.68, but changes year to year.

How they calculate your GPA: The GPA is calculated as a straight average. If you do not meet this average, the average of the last two years will be considered, with a cut-off of 3.78.

MCAT: Minimum of 10 in each section, with a "P" on the writing sample.

Personal: Mission statement: "To advance our tradition of preparing excellent physicians and leaders in healthcare, we embrace a spirit of inquiry and innovation in education and research."

Personal factors important to selection include: commitment, achievement, scientific reasoning and critical thinking, problem-solving and self-directed learning as well as "team player" skills, adaptability, creativity, extracurricular activities, evidence of the ability to cope with stress, communication skills, and sensitivity to others.

Letters of recommendation: Three letters of recommendation are required.

Invitation to interview: This is based on the cut-off criteria established for the MCAT and GPA. These vary from year to year.

Interview style: Unknown

Acceptance: After invitation for interview, it's a clean slate. Your offer of a seat will be based 50 percent on your interview, and 50 percent on your letters of recommendation and your personal information you provided with your application.

Curriculum description:

Year 1:

- The Cell, Genetics, and Neoplasia
- Energy Metabolism and Homeostasis
- Injury and Repair
- Inflammation Healing
- Neurotransmission Drugs and Receptors
- Musculoskeletal System
- Microbiology and Immunology
- Infectious Disease
- Oncology
- Dermatology
- Haematology

Concurrent courses:
- Medicine in Society
- Communication and Clinical Skills
- Anatomy

Year 2:

- Neurosciences
- Ophthalmology
- Otolaryngology
- Psychiatry
- Genitourinary
- Cardiovascular
- Respiratory

Concurrent courses:

- Medicine in Society

- Communication and Clinical Skills

Year 3:

- Endocrinology
- Reproduction/ Women's Health
- Gastrointestinal

Concurrent courses:

- Medicine in Society
- Communication and Clinical Skills

Year 4: Clinical clerkship:

- family medicine
- psychiatry
- paediatrics
- surgery
- obstetrics and gynaecology
- internal medicine
- emergency medicine anesthesiology
- elective time

Special programs or opportunities: Unknown

Information for special applicants:

Graduate students: As a graduate student, your degree must be completed before the commencement of medical school. You need to meet the MCAT cut-off but not the GPA cut-off. However, your grades from your undergraduate degree need to be "satisfactory," or show a trend of rising grades. If the graduate degree committee thinks you're suitable, you'll be invited to interview.

Aboriginal students: There's an alternative process for admission for up to four Aboriginal students per year. You need to include a letter of intent stating your Aboriginal affiliation and why you want to become a doctor. You are also required to submit a letter of support from your community. The GPA cut-off is 3.00 and the MCAT scores need to be 8 or better to receive an interview, except in exceptional circumstances.

Information source: http://www.normed.ca/ and http://www.ouac.on.ca/omsas/

Northern Ontario School of Medicine

Information source: http://www.normed.ca/ and http://www.ouac.on.ca/omsas/

Location: Thunder Bay and Sudbury, Ontario

Contact information:
http://www.normed.ca/
nomsadmit@normed.ca

West Campus
955 Oliver Rd
Thunder Bay, ON P7B 5E1
Tel: (807) 766-7300
Fax: (807) 766-7370

East Campus
935 Ramsey Lake Rd
Sudbury, ON P3E 2C6
Tel: (705) 675-4883
Fax: (705) 675-4858

Number of seats: 56

What are my chances? 1 in 37.5. Last available statistic stated 2,098 applications for 56 positions.

Duration of degree: 4 years

Tuition: $15,450

How do I apply? Apply through OMSAS
http://www.ouac.on.ca/omsas/

Application deadline: Register by September 15th, submit by October 3rd.

Admission Criteria

Number of credits: A 4-year undergraduate degree, unless applying as a mature student, meaning you're over 25. Mature students may apply with a 3-year degree.

Required courses: There are no required courses.

Required GPA: 3.00 on the 4.00 scale is required to apply. The average GPA of those interviewed is 3.6. The average of those accepted was 3.72 in 2006.
How they calculate your GPA: If you completed a 4-year degree before applying, the weight is as follows:

> 1st year=0
> 2nd year GPA x 1
> 3rd year GPA x 2
> 4th year GPA x 3
> then divide by 6

If you're in the process of completing a 4-year degree while you're applying, or if you're a mature student who has already completed a degree, the WGPA is calculated as:

> 1st year=0
> 2nd year GPA x 1
> 3rd year GPA x 2
> then divide by 3

If you're a mature student in the process of completing a 3-year degree, only your marks in your 2nd year are considered.

MCAT: Not required

Personal:

Guiding Values

- "a passion for living in, working in, and serving northern urban, rural, and remote communities"
- "sensitivity to diversity"
- "excellence in medical practice, teaching, learning, and professionalism"

Interest in the northern community and under-serviced populations, cross-cultural experiences, volunteer and extracurricular activities, and an ability to identify and fulfill community needs.

Letters of recommendation: Three are required. It's recommended that one is from someone in your community or an organization within your community.

Invitation to interview: Based on the weighted GPA and admissions questionnaire. About four hundred people are invited to interview.

Interview style: Multiple Mini Interview

Curriculum description:

Year 1:

- Northern and Rural Health
- Personal and Professional Aspects of Medical Practice
- Social and Population Health
- Foundations of Medicine
- Clinical Skills in Healthcare

There's a case-based approach during year one of the following topics:

- cardiovascular/respiratory system
- gastrointestinal system
- central and peripheral nervous system
- endocrine system
- musculo-skeletal system

Year 2:

- Northern and Rural Health
- Personal and Professional Aspects of Medical Practice
- Social and Population Health
- Foundations of Medicine
- Clinical Skills in Healthcare

There is a case-based approach during year two on the following topics:

- reproductive system
- renal system
- haematology/immunology
- neurological/behavioural
- end of life issues

Year 3:

comprehensive community clerkship:

Clerkship time with a family physician in a rural community while continuing with case-based problems.

Year 4:

Clerkship in core rotations of:
- surgery
- medicine
- woman's health
- mental health
- children's health

Information for special applicants:

Graduate students: There's no separate application for people with a masters or PhD. You still need to meet the requirement of four years of undergraduate education with a weighted GPA of at least 3.0. However, if you've completed graduate work, 0.2 will be added to your weighted GPA. This new WGPA will be used in the application process. You must finish your graduate degree by September of the year you're applying

Applicants who possess a graduate degree (masters or PhD) are not considered for admission as part of a separate applicant pool. All applicants are assessed for admission consideration based on the minimum requirement of a 4-year recognized undergraduate university degree (3-year degree for mature applicants) with a minimum WGPA of 3.0 on the 4.0 scale. Please see question #5 for WGPA details.

After the initial calculation is done to ensure compliance with the cut-off, an additional 0.2 will be added to the weighted GPA for the next stage in the application screening process. For example, if your weighted GPA is 3.3, your final weighted GPA for consideration will be 3.5.

You need to provide a letter from your graduate program stating that they're aware that you're applying to medical school. You'll also need to submit a final transcript by December of the year you're applying to medical school.

Aboriginal students: There are two seats reserved specifically for Aboriginal students. To apply through the Aboriginal stream, you are required to have a letter of support mailed directly to the school from your community.

University of Ottawa, Faculty of Medicine

Information source: http://www.medicine.uottawa.ca/eng/ and http://www.ouac.on.ca/omsas/

Location: Ottawa, Ontario

Contact information:
Admissions
Faculty of Medicine
University of Ottawa
451 Smyth Road, Room 2046
Ottawa, ON K1H 8M5
Tel: (613) 562-5409
Fax: (613) 562-5651
E-mail: admissM.D.@uottawa.ca

Number of seats: 123

What are my chances? 1 in 25.7. There are 3,161 applicants for 123 seats.

Duration of degree: 4 years

Tuition: Unknown

How do I apply? Apply through OMSAS
http://www.ouac.on.ca/omsas/

Application deadline: Register by September 15th, submit by October 3rd.

Admission Criteria

Number of credits: Three years of full-time studies in any program.

Required courses: 1 year of biology including a lab, 1 full year of humanities or social science. 2 full-year courses of chemistry, choosing from general biochemistry without a lab, general chemistry with a lab, or organic chemistry with a lab.

Required GPA: The required GPA is different for each geographical area.

How they calculate your GPA: Weighted GPA based on three most recent years of grades, with the most recent year weighted more heavily: The last three years of undergraduate grades are used for the WGPA calculation. The most recent year x3, the next most recent year x2, and the least recent year x1.

e.g., Year 3 GPA 3.5 x3 = 10.5
      Year 2 GPA 3.2 x2= 6.4
      Year 1 GPA 3.5 x1 = 3.5
      (10.5 + 6.4 + 3.5) /6 = 3.4

If you've only completed 2 years at the time of application, then the most recent year is weighted x2, and the next most recent year x1

e.g., Year 2 GPA 3.6 x2 = 7.2
   Year 1 GPA 3.4 x1= 3.4
   (7.2 +3.4)/3 = 3.53

If you've completed more than three years of marks when you're applying, you eliminate the least recent years of study.

e.g., GPA year 5= 3.4 x3 = 10.2
   GPA year 4= 3.7 x2 = 7.4
   GPA year 3= 3.5 x1 = 3.5
   GAP year 2= 3.2 à eliminate from calculation
   GPA year 1= 3.3l à eliminate from calculation
   (10.2 + 7.2 +3.5)/6 = 3.48

MCAT: MCAT is not required

Personal: The medical program emphasises self-learning. The program also focuses on teaching trust, communication skills, compassion, and ethics. Only activities since the beginning of university will be taken into account. When expanding on activities emphasise why you chose the activity, what you gained
from it, and how it will prepare you to be a future physician.

Letters of recommendation: Three letters of recommendation are required.
Invitation to interview: If your weighted GPA meets cut-off, your application will be further evaluated by means of your personal autobiographical sketch.
From this group, 500 people will be invited to interview at the University of Ottawa.

Interview style: Interviews are conducted in either English or French, depending on the choice of language of instruction of the applicant.

Curriculum description:

Year 1:

- Development and Homeostasis
- Hemotology and Neoplasia
- Cardiovascular

- Respiratory
- Renal
- Physician Skills Development I
- Infection and Host Response

Year 2:

- Endocrinology
- Human Reproduction and Sexuality
- Muscoloskeletal
- Neurology
- Mind
- Special Senses
- Gastrointestinal
- Physician Skills Development 2

Clerkship:

- link period
- surgery
- medicine
- obstetrics and gynaecology
- paediatrics
- psychiatry
- ambulatory medicine
- family medicine
- acute care medicine

Special programs or opportunities: Unknown.

Information for special applicants:

Graduate students: You're still required to complete all of the undergraduate pre-requisite courses. You can only apply if y finished or are in the last year of your graduate degree. A masters or a two-year PhD doesn't count. If your unde meet the WGPA cut-off, then there's no special for If they don't, you need to meet these basic require

If you're applying as a francophone or person of aboriginal ancestry, then you need an undergrad GPA of 3.30. If you're applying to the Anglophone pool, you require an undergrad GPA of 3.5. If you meet these criteria, then the grades acquired in year one of a course-based graduate program will count as the final year when calculating the WGPA.

You need to have maintained an A average during the graduate degree. Your productivity during the degree will then be evaluated.

McGill University Faculty of Medicine

Information source: http://www.medicine.mcgill.ca/ugme/

Location: Montreal, Quebec

Contact information:
Faculty of Medicine Admissions Office
McGill University
Suite 602
3655 Sir William Osler Promenade
Montreal, Quebec H3G 1Y6 CANADA
Telephone: +1 (514) 398-3517
Fax: +1 (514) 398-4631
Email: admissions.med @mcgill .ca
http://www.medicine.mcgill.ca/ugme/
Number of seats: 172

ed for Québec residents.
ents.

ou've
one-year
graduate marks
mula for your marks.
ents.

aculty of Medicine Home Page.

ns/applying/applynow_en.htm

Application deadline: Nov 15th, unless you're a resident of Quebec, giving you until Jan 15th.

Admission Criteria

Number of Credits: 120 credits (4 years full course load)
      6 credits general/introductory biology
      6 credits general/introductory chemistry
      6 credits general/introductory physics
      3 credits introductory organic chemistry

Courses in biochemistry, cell biology, and molecular biology are recommended but not mandatory.

Required GPA: Minimum of 3.5 on a 4.0 scale to be competitive - a recent mean GPA of accepted applicants was 3.74.
How they calculate your GPA: This is calculated as the straight average of your undergraduate courses.

MCAT: The MCAT is required. A minimum score of 30 with 8 as the lowest score in any one section. A recent average profile of accepted applicants is as follows:
VR 9.6
PS 11.2
BS 11.5
Overall score 32.26.

Personal: An autobiographical letter is submitted. This letter should explain the characteristics of the applicant and why they would make a good doctor. The committee is interested in examples of empathy, compassion and service to others, leadership, initiative, originality, the ability for good communication, the ability to work alone, and the ability to interact positively with others.

Letters of recommendation: Three letters of recommendation, with at least one or two of them coming from faculty.

Invitation to interview: This is based on your GPA, MCAT scores, and personal characteristics.

Interview style: At least two interviews in a one-on-one basis with members of the admissions committee.

Curriculum description:

Year 1 (includes first half of year 2)

- Basis of Medicine
- Molecules, Cells, and Tissues
- Gases, Fluids, and Electrolytes
- Life Cycle
- Endocrinology, Metabolism, and Nutrition
- Nervous System and Special Senses
- Host Defence and Host Paracite
- Pathobiology, treatment, and prevention of disease

Year 2 (second half only)

- Introduction to Clinical Medicine (ICM)
- Ethics and Health Law
- Intro to Internal Medicine, Pediatrics, Surgery, Anesthesia, Opthalmology, Family Medicine, Oncology, Neurology, Radiology, Dermatology and Psychiatry

Year 3:
Clerkship:
- rural family medicine
- urban family medicine
- medicine
- obstetrics and gynecolcogy
- general surgery
- paediatrics
- psychiatry
- emergency medicine
- elective

Year 4:

Senior Clerkships:

- geriatrics

- surgery sub-specialties
- medicine and society
- topics in medical science
- electives

Special programs or opportunities: **M.D./PhD and M.D./MBA**

Information for special applicants:

Graduate students: There's no separate stream for those with a graduate degree. There's no advantage to your GPA. However, a graduate degree will be considered a "Professional Accomplishment."

Aboriginal students: Aboriginal students are invited to apply.

Information source: http://www.medicine.dal.ca/

Dalhousie University Faculty of Medicine

Information source: http://www.medicine.dal.ca/

Location: Halifax, Nova Scotia
Contact information:
Room C-125 - Clinical Research Centre - 5849 University Avenue
Dalhousie University - Halifax, NS B3H 4H7
Tel 902-494-1546 - Fax 902-494-8884
http://www.medicine.dal.ca/

Number of seats: 90 total. 81 seats are reserved for maritime students, 9 for out-of-province students.

What are my chances? 90% of seats are reserved for applicants from the Maritimes. For the out-of-province applicants, Dalhousie recently received 440 applications for 9 seats, making the chances for an out-of-province applicant about 1 in 50.

Duration of degree: 4 years

Tuition: Unknown

How do I apply? Download the application from the Dalhousie website, and mail it in.

Application deadline: postmarked by October 31st.

Admission Criteria

Number of credits: In the final year of a four-year degree (preferably), although sometimes an applicant with a three-year degree is considered.

Required courses: No specific courses are required. However, taking two or three science classes at a challenging level is suggested.
Required GPA: Maritime applicants: minimum GPA of 3.3 on a 4.3 scale, and non-maritime applicants: minimum of 3.7 on a 4.3 scale.

How they calculate your GPA: Straight average.

MCAT: Maritime applicants: total score of 24, 8 in each of PS, BS, and VR. One score of 7 is acceptable, but the total still has to be 24 non-maritime applicants: total score of 30 with a 10 in each of PS, BS, and VR. One 9 can be achieved as long as the total score is 30.

Personal:
Mission Statement: "The Faculty of Medicine, Dalhousie University, strives to benefit society through equal commitment to exemplary patient care, education, and the discovery and advancement of knowledge. We aim to create and maintain a learning and research environment of national and international stature, enabling our graduates and us to serve the health needs of the Maritime Provinces and Canada."

Essay: An opportunity for you to express your views and describe your strengths and weaknesses. The committee is interested in leadership, volunteer, and community service experience. Experiences that demonstrate your emotional stability, maturity and communication skills, your curiosity, social values, initiative, and reliability are considered beneficial when assessing non-academic factors.

Letters of recommendation: Three letters of reference.

Invitation to interview: All candidates with "a reasonable chance of admission" are interviewed.

Interview style: Interviewed by two people, either a medical student and a faculty member, or two faculty members.

Curriculum description:

Year 1:

- Human Body
- Metabolism & Function
- Pathology, Immunology & Microbiology
- Pharmacology
- Genetics, Embryology, and Reproduction

Longitudinal courses:
- Clinical Epidemiology & Critical Thinking
- Patient-Doctor
- Electives

Year 2:

- Brain and Behaviour
- Skin, Glands and Blood
- Cardiovascular and Respiratory
- Genitourinary, Gastrointestinal and Musculoskeletal

Longitudinal Courses:

- Population Health, Community Service & Critical Thinking
- Patient - Doctor
- Elective

Years 3 and 4, Clerkship:

Introduction to the Clerkship

- family medicine

- psychiatry
- obstetrics and gynaecology
- paediatrics
- internal medicine
- surgical
- emergency medicines
- continuing & preventive care
- care of the elderly
- electives

Special programs or opportunities: Unknown

Information for special applicants:

Graduate students: The thesis must be submitted prior to starting medical school. The acceptability of the course load is decided on a case-by case basis.

Faculty of Medicine, Memorial University of Newfoundland

Information source: http://www.med.mun.ca/
Location: St. John's, Newfoundland

Contact information:
Admissions Office
Faculty of Medicine
Memorial University of Newfoundland
Room 1751, Health Sciences Centre
St. John's, NL Canada, A1B 3V6
Telephone: (709) 777-6615
Fax: (709) 777-8422
Email: munmed@mun.ca

Number of seats: 60

What are my chances? 1 in 12.5. There are about 750 applications for the 60 available seats. 67% of seats are reserved for residents of Newfoundland and Labrador, 16% for residents of New Brunswick, and

3% for residents of Prince Edward Island. 7% are for residents from other provinces in Canada, and 7% are reserved for international applicants.

Duration of degree: 4 years

Tuition: $6,250

How do I apply? Online at http://www.med.mun.ca/admissions/

Application deadline: Mid-October

Admission Criteria

Number of credits: A four-year undergraduate degree.

Required courses: Two semesters of English (AP, Ontario OAC, 4 English courses at CEGEP, International Baccalaureate Programme English courses may be considered as equivalent). It's suggested (although not mandatory) that basic physical and life sciences courses may be helpful for writing the MCAT and in preparing for medicine.

Required GPA: Approximately 80%.

How they calculate your GPA: Straight average of all courses taken, including graduate courses.

MCAT: The Average MCATs of previous years were 9's on each section and an O in the writing sample section.

Personal:

Mission Statement: "Our purpose is to enhance the health of the people of Newfoundland and Labrador by educating physicians and health scientists; by conducting research in clinical and basic medical sciences and applied health sciences and by promoting the skills and attitudes of lifelong learning."

Personal characteristics: Maturity, self-evaluation skills, attitudes towards society, leadership, dependability, personal insight, adaptability, empathy, compassion, and communication skills. Work experience, extracurricular activities, volunteer work, sports activities, health-elated activities and community involvement are taken into consideration to help evaluate these characteristics.

Letters of recommendation: Two, with at least one of them being an academic recommendation.

Invitation to interview: Unknown

Interview style: Interview lasts approximately one hour with two interviewers.

Curriculum description:

Years 1 and 2:

- Basic Science of Medicine (an integrated course including biochemistry, physiology, immunology, cell biology, genetics, microbiology, nutrition, pharmacology, pathology and anatomy)
- Clinical Skills
- Community Health
- Integrated Study of Disease
- Family Medicine Preclerkship Elective

Years 3 and 4, Clerkship:

- clerkship preparation course
- internal medicine
- surgery
- psychiatry
- paediatrics
- rural family practice
- obstetrics/gynaecology
- elective time
- selective time
- Integrated Basic, Community Health, and Clinical Sciences

Special programs or opportunities: M.D./PhD

Information for special applicants:

Graduate students: All marks earned in graduate school are included in your GPA. There's no special preference for graduate students.

APPENDIX A: ORGANIZING YOUR APPLICATIONS – A SAMPLE METHOD

GRADES

1st Year Subjects	Grade	Weight
Average		

2nd Year Subjects	Grade	Weight
Average		

3rd Year Subjects	Grade	Weight
Average		

GPA CHART

School	Formula	My GPA

MCAT: PS____ BS_____ VR_____ WS_____

School	AAMC #

UNIVERSITY TRANSCRIPTS

	School Attended	School attended
Medical School		
Medical School		
Medical School		

CV VERIFIERS

Activity	Year	Duration	Contact Name	Contact Number

REFERENCE LETTER WRITERS

Name	Position	For Which Schools?	Ask?	CV?	Meeting?	Currier?

PERSONAL STATEMENT

Medical School	Personal Statement Written?

APPENDIX B: SAMPLE INTERVIEW QUESTIONS

Here is a set of questions that might be asked of you on interview day. Some of these are from personal experience; some are from what others have told me they were asked; some I made up; some are from the following websites that I encourage you to visit:

http://www.studentdoctor.net/interview/index.asp
http://www.mymedline.com/premed/int_sampleqa.php3
http://career.berkeley.edu/Health/MedInterview.stm
http://www.essayedge.com/medical/admissions/interview.shtml
http://zoology.muohio.edu/premed/Interview.html
http://www.agriculture.purdue.edu/anscjobs/medical/questions.pdf

Sample Questions

Tell me about a problem that you wish you'd handled differently.

Imagine you're working as a resident in a hospital. What role do you see yourself fulfilling as a part of this kind of team?

What's the biggest challenge in healthcare today? How do we solve it?

What personal quality do you think you'll have to work the hardest to improve during your medical school experience?

What would make you decide to stop studying medicine?

What does *quality of life* mean?

How do you respond when a group member isn't pulling their weight?

Some people think that the new or younger generation of physicians are not as hard-working (i.e., wanting to leave right at 5:00 p.m., not wanting to put in as long of a work-week). How do you feel about this perception?

Are you tough?

In what situations have you been judgmental?

Do you feel there's too much emphasis on prevention in medicine?

Why do you want to become a doctor?

What would be your biggest fear in practicing medicine?

What makes a good doctor? What makes a dangerous doctor?

Tell me something to make me laugh.

Why haven't you contributed your service towards your undergraduate school instead of other volunteer work?

Discuss a healthcare issue that's been in the news in the past month.

Do you think doctors make too much money?

What kind of health problems would you encounter if you were practicing up north with a native population?

What are some leadership positions you've had?

What qualities do you look for in a team member?

Tell me about your research.

What are the community implications of a needle-exchange program? Can you think of any alternatives?

What are the social implications of gambling?

What would your solution be to the doctor shortage in rural areas?

Who's your role model?

How do you balance your time?

Would you feel guilty for going overseas to provide healthcare while many of your fellow Canadians are waiting months and months to be seen by a doctor?

What do you think will be the biggest problem facing medicine in five years, ten years, in twenty years?

Describe an ethical situation that you may encounter in the medical profession and how you'd handle it.

Describe a decision you regret making and why.

What would you do if a peer in your class seemed depressed or suicidal?

You're part of the Healthcare Budget Committee. Decide where the money for healthcare is spent.

What's your opinion on two-tier healthcare?

How would you tell the parents of a young child that their child was terminally ill with cancer?

What event in the world's history do you think has had the greatest impact on today's society?

How do you plan to balance your personal life with being a doctor?

If your schedule was totally cleared for one day, what would you do to pass the time?

Describe your support system.

Can you think of a time that you made a mistake but it ended up working out better because of it?

Prove to me that you have compassion.

Give me an example of when you failed.

Tell me of a time you were truly altruistic. Is it possible to be truly altruistic? Does it matter?

If you could recommend one book for the whole world to read what would it be?

If your father was ill and on a waitlist, would you drive to Buffalo for diagnostic treatment?

If you could change one aspect of your character what would it be?

How do you deal with boredom?

Prove to me you know how to manage your time.

What was the most painful emotional experience you've ever had? How did you cope with it?

What would you do if you saw a co-worker steal medication?

What do you think about nurse practitioners?

Suppose you were a medical student and you detected alcohol on the breath of your supervisor (who can make or break you). What would you do?

Can you think of a situation when you displayed the qualities of a physician, a situation where you didn't, and what you learned from them?

You're on duty in the ER when an unconscious three-year-old girl is brought in. It's clear that she needs an immediate blood transfusion to survive, but her Jehovah's Witness parents are adamantly against it. What would you do and why?

A senior citizen is suffering from terminal cancer and is in continuous agony despite being given high doses of painkillers. He asks you, his primary doctor, to euthanize him, saying: "I've always made my own decisions and have been responsible for them. I want to die with dignity." What would you do and why?

Is it ever okay for a doctor to give false hope?

Who has influenced you the most?

When would you prescribe birth control to a twelve-year-old?

What do you think about alternative medicine and what would you do if your patient told you they were also seeing a naturopath?

What are the negative aspects of being a doctor?

Define integrity.

Why are you applying to medicine and not another healthcare profession?

Why don't you want to be a nurse?

Don't you think you could help more people if you continued on in your graduate studies and made a major breakthrough in your field, rather than becoming a doctor?

What makes you sure you can handle the workload of a physician?

How do you feel about the conflict in the Middle East?

How do you feel about the current Canadian prime minister?

Your young female patient wants a genetic test to see if she has the breast cancer gene, but her mother does not want her to have the test because if it's positive it might mean she has it too. What do you do?

If you had ten million dollars to spend in the healthcare sector, where would you spend it?

Tell us about a time when you completely changed your point-of-view on a long-held opinion.

Name a time when you dropped the ball and why.

You're a fifty-year-old diabetic woman who's functionally impaired and just out of insulin. How do you feel?

You are a patient addicted to opiates and you just found out you were put on a six-month waiting list before you can start a rehabilitation program. How do you feel?

How do you feel about affirmative action in the United States?

How will you feel if you go to medical school and you're only an average student there?

What's the most important lessons your parents taught you?

Am I entitled to healthcare if I'm a smoker who does not want to quit?

Am I entitled to healthcare if I'm obese and I choose not to exercise?

How would you explain to a small child why it rains?

What role do you see clinical trials playing in your research?

How do you reconcile your very broad range of interests with a career in medicine?

What will you do if you're not accepted into medical school?

Think of an ethical situation and discuss both sides of the issue.

Why do you think mental illness has stigma?

Comment on one group of people in Canada requiring specialized and distinct healthcare.

What would you do if your mother was diagnosed with a terminal illness around the same time as your final medical school examinations?

Do you think that doctors have too much or too little power?

APPENDIX C: ALTERNATIVE CAREERS

Audiology and Speech Language Pathology

http://www.caslpa.ca/

Chiropody

http://www.ontariochiropodist.com/

Dentistry

http://www.cda-adc.ca/

Dietician

http://www.dietitians.ca/

Genetic Counselling

http://www.cagc-accg.ca/section/view/

Midwifery

http://www.canadianmidwives.org/

Nursing

http://www.cna-nurses.ca/cna/

Occupational Therapy

http://www.caot.ca/

Physiotherapy

http://www.physiotherapy.ca/

Psychologist

http://www.cpa.ca/

Respiratory Therapist

http://www.csrt.com/about.php?display&en&23

Ultrasonographer

http://www.cardup.org/

Veterinary Medicine

http://canadianveterinarians.net/index.aspx

X-ray Technician

http://www.camrt.ca/

APPENDIX D: SAMPLE MEDICAL SCHOOL APPLICATION LETTERS

Sample 1

My palms were sweating and my face was beet red. Standing in front of my ninth-grade class to read an essay out loud, I cursed that my pasty white complexion was forever giving away my embarrassment. The assignment was simple—to give a speech on the topic of your choice. Hearing this, my heart sank, and I decided to ask the teacher for an alternate assignment. She allowed me to write an essay instead, but I still had to read it in front of the class. I chose the topic of Down's syndrome and used the example of a boy named Tristan, whose spirit touched many hearts and who's life is recorded in a book of his own name. Something interesting happened as I was reading through the essay in front of my classmates. I found myself slowly forgetting that they were even there. The topic was so fascinating and Tristan's story so inspiring, I became excited about what I had written. This was the first time I forgot my fear of public speaking and simply expressed myself. It was an important step in realizing, too, that I was putting too much stock in what others thought of me. The war was not over but that day, in ninth-grade, I had won a battle.

Fast-forward five years. Along with several volunteers, I worked at a hospital and health development agency in rural Honduras. To pass the time in the small, rural village, we would often have evenings of camaraderie when we would share stories about our home countries. As the volunteers were from all over the world, and many of the local villagers wished they could travel, we always found a lot to talk about. We took turns hosting the evenings and, inevitably, it was my turn. How was I supposed to present what it means to be Canadian? And in Spanish, no less?! I was wracked with nervousness. As I begun my presentation, however, I realized with surprise that I was having fun. These people didn't care that my Spanish was broken, or that I seemed a little silly demonstrating such absurdities as fishing beneath the *ice,* of all things! I dug deep and came up with descriptions of ice-fishing, grizzly bears, and maple syrup. I even got the room playing the French-Canadian spoons to the tunes of Maritimer, Ashley MacIsaac! Once again, I had taken another step in overcoming the personal challenge of public speaking. I was happy about how the evening had turned out, but little did I know, the toughest part of overcoming this fear was yet to come.

It was the fourth year of my undergraduate degree. I had not slept a wink all weekend. On Monday, I was going to give my first of five presentations in a physiology seminar course. I had to study a scientific paper and present it in a professional format to other students and three professors. I had never even heard of a Western Blot, and the definition of an ANOVA statistic was buried beneath a few years of dust! I was far from comfortable with the vocabulary of the field and was convinced the other students would laugh at me. Monday came and my presentation, though mediocre, was a starting point. I was nervous and it showed. I did, however, get praise for my interest in the subject matter and for my overhead materials. It was not a total loss! Over the semester, I gradually improved. My confidence in the material grew, as did my familiarity with reading scientific papers. I reminded myself that the purpose of education was to learn and to improve, and I became less influenced by the opinions of my peers. At the end of the semester, I had been ridden with anxiety and sleep-deprivation, but I would not have changed a thing. I had improved tremendously and grown so much from the challenge of these experiences. I had faced my silent demon.

Speaking in front of others has been a lifelong battle, but I am consciously facing each opportunity to overcome this fear. I know that I stand only to gain. Since my seminar course, I have given an address at city hall, emceed an arts festival at a local theatre, and given a presentation to my graduate committee. I am far from being over my fear of public speaking, but I have come to learn that to develop such a skill only stands to benefit me. The biggest obstacles are within ourselves and I often remind myself of a quotation I once heard. "We wouldn't care so much about what people thought of us, if only we realized how little they did!"

Sample 2

Many things influence a person over the course of their life: people, events, tragedies, and accomplishments. The sum of these occurrences, along with family and heredity, create the individual. Several major events and people have helped structure who I am at this point in my life. As I grow older, I change and mature with each added experience. I feel that in order to introduce myself, it is not sufficient to describe who I am, and therefore must narrate how I've become the person I am today.

Events early in life mold an individual, but I will not claim to remember which incidences were significant for me as a child. I can, however, explain which events I feel built my character within the last several years. In the summer of 1995 I went on an Outward Bound trip into the coastal mountain range of B.C. Outward Bound is a program that leads ten young people out into the wilderness for a total of twenty-one days for a lesson in survival and nature appreciation. The course includes a three-day solo camp, rock climbing, ice climbing, navigation, and non-intrusive mountaineering. It challenged me to overcome my fears of the wilderness and become comfortable with skills that I had just learned. I had to learn to deal with the problem of lacking what I had considered to be the everyday essentials (e.g., shower, bathroom, and fresh food), which in turn led me to fully appreciate the conveniences that we have in modern society. I feel the experience made me grow quickly, since I had to learn how to deal with different people in tense situations. It taught me to think clearly in times of stress and to believe in my own skills, but also to recognize my own limitations. The final outcome of the course was to turn a group of teenagers into conscientious young adults with wilderness skills, and more importantly, with confidence and goals.

I also had the opportunity to participate in the Science One Program. This program, which I participated in during the 1996-1997 school year, is designed to integrate the basic sciences into one coherent course. The professors promote independent learning and thought, and the course is aimed to hone the students' problem solving and basic logic skills. I found this course to be a challenge when coming out of high school since it required more than just memory work and simple analysis. The difference in the teaching atmosphere, along with the new experiences of university life and living away from home, caused my first year to be very difficult and un-enjoyable. However, over the course of the year, I learned how to study and how to learn. I became aware of the constant interactions of all the science disciplines and realized the need for proper time management. I learned organization skills that help in all aspects of my life, and at the end of the school year, I became the president of the Science One Society. Becoming the president of this society was great because it allowed me to help younger students deal with the same problems that I had had the previous year.

Many other experiences also contributed to the person I have become. I continued to want to help younger students and became an Imagine University group leader. I taught, participated in swing dancing, founded a University Improv Theatre society, went to New York for two weeks, achieving my black belt in tae kwon do, volunteering in the ER and researching my undergraduate thesis. Each event has taught me an important lesson about life and people. Some events have taught me how to be a good leader, while others have provided me with the help numerous people. I have had ample opportunity to teach, to coach, and to learn because I was willing to invest my time and effort into these various activities.

I believe that everyone in a person's life in some way affects who they become, through teaching, arguing, playing, and many other possible interactions. Yet, with all this feedback, there still remain several key figures who have had greater influence than others. There are three people in my life who I see as major contributors to my character. The first is my mother, who has been a positive role model throughout my life. Here I am not simply referring to the stereotypical image of a mother; I specifically mean my mother's personality. She had a very difficult life—lack of money, moving to a new country, escape from communism and anti-Semitism—yet through all of this she remains the most positive, optimistic person I have ever met. She is always encouraging and looks at the lighter side of life, claiming that if she didn't, she would have gone mad many years ago. The second major contributor is my brother. My brother is twelve years older than I, and has always been a role model for me. The reason I claim that my brother has been a positive role model is that he constantly makes me question everything. Every idea I possess or passing impulse that I get has to overcome an extensive array of questions from him. He makes me think about life, love, the future, religion, and any other issue that you may be inclined to name. He motivates me by arguing with me and playing the antagonist. The third influence is my Outward Bound instructor. He affected me in two ways. First, my life was in his hands for the duration of the course—three weeks—and I grew very trusting of him. Second, he showed me that I must strive towards any goals that I set for myself. He was a very talented musician and academic, yet chose to leave the conveniences of the modern world for the ruggedness of a tent and a sleeping bag. He spent all of his time teaching Outward Bound courses and was therefore always in the wilderness. He showed me that it was acceptable not to know what I wanted to do in life, but that when I found out, I must pursue my goals with enthusiasm.

I am a hard working, confident individual. I am intelligent, charismatic and outgoing. I put a lot of emphasis on school work and self-directed learning, yet remain well rounded and involved in the community and in social events. I deal well with people and want the ability and means to help them. I am honest and display many leadership qualities, including listening, mediating, and organizing. I enjoy many different activities such as dancing, scuba diving, theatre, sports, and travelling. Medicine has always appealed to me and I strive to be a physician for a number of reasons. First, the life sciences have always interested me and medicine remains a dynamic field to which one must constantly adapt. Second, this career would allow me to meet and interact with numerous people from different background and cultures. I have found that I am a social person and enjoy dealing with and helping as many people as I can. Third, physicians are needed all around the world and this career ensures job stability and job freedom. A physician takes on the role of caregiver, friend, and mentor. I believe I have the skills and responsibility to take on this daunting task, and would make an excellent doctor.

Sample 3

There we were, a group of fifteen fishers, researchers, technicians, and students, seated in a circle in the conference room of the Coast Guard vessel, the *Martha Black*. We were participating in a deep-sea coral research expedition in the Northeast Channel, a large underwater inlet off the South Shore of Nova Scotia. The head scientist was explaining how the remotely operated vehicle, the ROPOS, was going to function and how a single researcher on the deck of the boat would guide the submersible through the depths and forests of corals one kilometre below the surface.

I participated in the expedition as part of a Natural Sciences and Engineering Research Council-funded independent research project on the morphology and distribution of Nova Scotia's deep sea corals in the summer of 2001.

While there has always been a general recognition of the importance of coral reefs among certain fishing industries, general public interest and awareness of deep-sea corals and their ecological, economic and social significance are not as widely held. Thus, the principle purpose of my research project was to collate information gathered from a variety of sources and stakeholders, including scientific journals, century-old catalogues from the first deep-sea research cruises, and personal interviews with fishers and natural museum curators.

My time on the boat was both physically and mentally challenging. Being of small stature, I was easily affected by the rocking motion of the ship and often suffered from bouts of seasickness despite the precautions I had taken before boarding. As all on board wanted to ensure that our time was not wasted, we worked incredibly long and tiring hours; we stopped only briefly for meals. Mentally, this project tested every person's ability to withstand a long stretch of time in small, closed quarters, in the middle of the ocean with no land in sight. It was daunting to think of the immensity of the ocean and how small the boat was. It was truly a humbling experience.

The challenges that this project offered and my ability to meet those challenges made my experiences working on corals and my time on the Coast Guard vessel among the most educational and enjoyable of my life. Prior to this study, I did not have the opportunity to conduct research in a self-directed and independent manner. This project, however, allowed me to take the necessary steps and initiative to collect all relevant information, network, meet with stakeholders and academics, conduct interviews, and ultimately to ensure deadlines were met. While such tasks were sometimes difficult, I found that keeping a positive attitude and a sense of humour helped to increase my confidence in my abilities and made the project progress more smoothly. I realised that it was important not to become anxious over the strict and looming deadlines and that ultimately, the project would be completed more effectively and efficiently if I remained composed and relaxed. I also met the challenges posed by both the project and the work being conducted on the Coast Guard ship by being able to adapt to the new situations that each day presented, by having an open mind and being patient.

Meeting the challenges of this project brought tangible results. I was able to successfully complete the first coral identification guide to have ever been published. More importantly, it has been distributed to fishers in the Maritimes with the hope that they will become more aware and conscious of the corals and the need to conserve them. I also continued my work on coral the following year when I wrote an independent report on the growth of corals on deep-sea telecommunication cables. This area of research has only begun to be studied by the scientific community and we hope to publish this report.

Of all my experiences, this one has most prepared me for the challenges that medical school, and ultimately being a physician, will hold. I know I will enjoy meeting the challenges that a career in medicine entails; those that are academic and are based on the actual study of the science, those that are technical and involve learning how to perform medical procedures, and those that are mental and require managing the stress that is inherent to the profession. I recognise the rigours of the medical school training program and the life-long commitment to learning that entering this program entails. It is, perhaps, in part because of this that I am eager to take on such challenges. Studying medicine and becoming a physician would not only be rewarding, it would also be a great privilege.

Sample 4

One of my strengths is that I am a highly motivated individual with a strong desire to learn outside of formal class time. My experiences in a physiology lab as a worker for Regional Residential Services Society (RRSS), a non-profit organization dedicated to helping individuals with intellectual disabilities, and my pursuits in the equestrian world demonstrate my high level of motivation. Through RRSS I have worked in both group and small-option homes and participated in several training seminars that have focused directly on developing communication skills with intellectually challenged people. This work has given me a chance to further explore my suitability as a physician by placing me one-on-one with people that require varying levels of counselling and medical care. My work in the physiology lab demonstrates my desire to learn outside of formal class time as I have studied to become familiar with the research and experimental techniques specific to ion channels and human disease.

A weakness I see in myself is that I often avoid confrontation. I tend to be quiet in nature; while this helps me as a listener, it impacts negatively on my ability to convey my ideas to others. I have been improving upon this weakness through participation in courses that have required work in small collaborative groups, thus allowing me to become more effective at expressing my ideas. Further practice in a small group setting will solidify my communication skills and help me to improve upon my ability to express my ideas and opinions towards others.

It has taken me some time to decide what I truly want to do with my life, which many may also see as a significant weakness. With the diversity of my interests, I have found it very difficult to focus directly on any single discipline. However, I have traveled around the world, lived in different cultures, and taken the time to learn deeply about who I am. It is impossible to find this kind of experience within the confines of a classroom, and through my experience, I have become more focused and more driven towards the goals I have set out to achieve.

Although I have not always wanted to become a physician, it is a goal to which I am now committed. By taking the time to explore the world, and ultimately my own strengths and desires, and by demonstrating my commitment towards helping the sick through work and volunteering, there will be no question down the road that deciding to enter medical school was the right decision. This will further strengthen my commitment to the patients I will eventually treat and my passion for the field. My interest in becoming a community leader and my genuine empathy for people in need will ensure my success as a physician and make me a good candidate for entrance into medicine.

ABOUT THE AUTHOR

Anne Berndl received her M.D. from McMaster University in 2005 and is currently pursuing specialty training as a resident in Obstetrics and Gynecology through Dalhousie University. In 2006, she was named "Top 30 under 30" in Halifax by the Halifax Daily News.

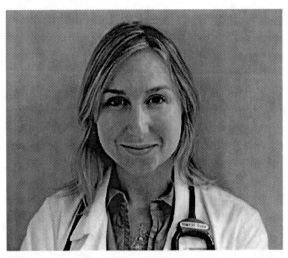

She completed a BSc.H. from Queen's University in 2002, during which she participated in research projects both at Queen's and though St. Michael's Hospital in Toronto. During university, Berndl spent a summer in rural Mexico participating in a cultural emersion program, was a Girl Guide Leader, a member of the Queen's Dance Club and was an actor in the university production of "The Vagina Monologues." On weekends, she worked at a foster home for children with disabilities. She also spent a few summers as a host at the Ontario Science Centre, where she lead nature walks and made paper out of elephant dung.

During high school, Berndl took her senior English credit at Oxford University and her senior Science credits at the Ontario Science Centre Science School. She was a member of the Improv team and Debating team, and participated in swimming, cross country and downhill skiing. She took Jazz and Ballet after school.

Anne Berndl was born and raised in Toronto where she spent most of her time catching snakes in her backyard.

Writing on Stone Press is currently accepting manuscripts and query letters for non-fiction books. We are especially seeking authors for our Canadian Career Series in the professions of Accounting, Dentistry, Chiropractic, Education, Architect, Engineer, Veterinarian, and Pharmacist.

Please forward your inquiries to:
Writing on Stone Press
Box 259
Raymond, Alberta
T0K 2S0
or fax us at 403-752-4815

At Writing on Stone Press, we strive to produce quality books for our audiences. If you have noticed any errors in this publication, please let us know so that we can make any necessary corrections for future printings. Thank you.

Printed in the United States
91715LV00001B/1-99/A